DISEASE
AND ITS CONQUEST

DISEASE
AND ITS CONQUEST

By

G. T. HOLLIS

HON. M.A. (OXON.)
Editor, *Oxford Medical Publications*

With a Foreword by

MAURICE DAVIDSON

M.A., M.D., B.CH. (OXON.), F.R.C.P. (LOND.)
Consulting Physician to the Brompton Hospital for
Consumption and Diseases of the Chest, &c.

GEOFFREY CUMBERLEGE
OXFORD UNIVERSITY PRESS
LONDON   NEW YORK   TORONTO
1953

Oxford University Press, Amen House, London E.C. 4

GLASGOW NEW YORK TORONTO MELBOURNE WELLINGTON
BOMBAY CALCUTTA MADRAS KARACHI CAPE TOWN IBADAN

Geoffrey Cumberlege, Publisher to the University

PRINTED IN GREAT BRITAIN

FOREWORD

THE ignorance of the general public on technical matters is proverbial. While this is true, more or less, in regard to all avocations for the pursuit of which a special training is required, it seems to apply with particular force to Medicine. Even the most educated and intelligent among the public, who may have acquired a tolerable conception of many technical occupations, e.g. the Law, Banking, the Stock Exchange, and so forth, when it comes to any question concerning health and disease too often betray their lack of acquaintance with fundamental principles. The medical profession has sometimes been reproached for its failure to attempt to instruct the lay public, who still incline to view disease much as did their unenlightened forebears and to look upon the performances of their medical advisers as an extant instance of mumbo-jumbo.

To the demand for simple but reliable information this book is intended to provide an answer. That it does so in a manner which should satisfy any person capable of exercising fair and reasonable judgement is due to certain unusual features of its origin. First, the author is not himself a medical man; he can therefore more easily regard his subject through the spectacles of the lay public, and with a philosophic detachment of which few medical men today appear capable. Secondly, he has spent thirty years or more in the task of editing and publishing technical works on medicine, surgery, and their allied sciences, with whose vocabulary he is naturally as familiar as with the language of everyday life. Lastly, his book is written in a cultivated and temperate manner, with every regard for the niceties of English style that should appeal to readers of taste.

The combination of these three factors in the production

of the book has made it unique in that it gives the reader something which could not have been supplied by the vast majority of qualified medical men, and certainly not by any layman who lacked that intimate contact with medical science which has made the author a doyen of medical publishing.

This volume is not a medical compendium for the masses. It is a work of art intended for educated persons. It contains all the technical details necessary for those to whom it is addressed, and, which is equally important, it portrays in the delivery of its message a nobility of purpose and a charm of language that should attract the most eclectic of readers.

MAURICE DAVIDSON

LONDON W. 1
January 1953

CONTENTS

INTRODUCTION

FROM the beginning, man, a rational creature, must have pondered over the many ills which afflict the flesh. Some, no doubt, he found fairly easy to understand—the loss of a limb, the putting-out of an eye, the crushing-in of a skull. For there it was not difficult to see the connexion between cause and effect. His familiarity with animal bones and human skeletons would enable him to comprehend broken limbs. He would notice too that severe wounding was followed by loss of quantities of a red fluid which was evidently vital, for if enough was lost the victim died. And so on. Gradually a mass of lore accumulated from generation to generation, concerning what we now term 'surgical' accidents. But there remained a vast number of wholly unaccountable happenings: people lost certain faculties apparently without cause; their bodies showed strange changes; they sickened and died; sometimes these inexplicable events affected only individuals, sometimes entire communities. Primitive man, unable to solve this problem of 'medical' illness, postulated demoniac intervention and, for only remedy, attempted to propitiate the supposedly malignant influences. When we smile at his ignorance, let us reflect that there was a working partnership between magic and medicine until quite recent times, and even at the present day a less primitive magic dignified with a 'scientific' label has its adherents.

Gradually man developed a reasoning curiosity about the construction and working of his body, and by infinitely small steps attained an understanding of anatomy and physiology, and of the corollary subject, pathology, which deals with the changes disease works in the body. Experiments were performed (frequently on the experimenter's own person), and dead bodies were dissected. For a long time investigators could know only what their unaided vision could perceive, but by the invention of the microscope in the seventeenth century the minutest structures of the body became visible and hitherto imperceptible processes of disease could be discerned. Later, with the discovery of the micro-organisms responsible for many specific diseases (a result of the work of microbiologists from 1860 onwards), the science of bacteriology emerged. On the diagnostic side progress was no less marked. The physicians of old had relied solely upon their observation of the patient's general condition, with pulse-taking as almost their only aid to their clinical instinct. Then came 'percussion'—the tapping of various regions to elicit significant responses, and 'auscultation'—listening to and interpreting the sounds from the heart and lungs which the invention of the stethoscope later made a scientific technique. The clinical thermometer assisted the detection of illness. Chemical analysis of the body's secretions and excretions brought the precision of the laboratory into the consulting-room. Instruments of ever-increasing delicacy and accuracy were invented—ophthalmoscopes, cystoscopes, bronchoscopes, gastroscopes; X-rays laid bare the innermost secrets of the living body in health and disease; the electro-encephalograph amplified our knowledge of the brain as the electrocardiograph did of the heart. The electron microscope has augmented the magnification of the most powerful optical instruments almost as much as the latter did that of the simple lens. New sciences, and new branches of the older learning, have reinforced classical medicine—biochemistry, pharmacology, genetics, cytology, psychiatry, radiology, haematology, neurology, to name but a few.

The end of diagnosis is treatment. From the earliest days some attempts were made to treat illness; a rough kind of surgery was practised even in prehistoric times. Later, in 'medical' cases, incantations began to give way to medicinal treatment of a sort. Knowledge of the properties of various plants and minerals, often accidentally discovered, was gradually systematized and extended into a materia medica. Although many treatments were highly efficacious, for a long time they remained empirical; while men knew that poppy-juice soothed pain, cinchona bark relieved fever, or lemons cured scurvy, they did not understand why; nor did they conceive any methods of research (other than the traditional system of trial and error) which might rationalize or enlarge their knowledge. Not until the beginning of the nineteenth century had medicine any pretensions to be called a science. At the opening of that wonderful century, the medical profession was in a condition not greatly advanced beyond that of Tudor times; at its close it was in all essentials what it is today. What made this transformation possible, and what is often overlooked, is that not only the scientific, but the social bases of medicine were laid at this time. Among the most important of these were the vast improvement in the system of education for the profession begun more than a century ago, and the ever-increasing facilities for the training of students in every branch; the regulation of status of its members; the standards laid down by law for their conduct and also for the mutual protection of themselves and the public; and the extension of legislation into the field of public health.

As even a bare list of the comparatively recent achievements of medicine would occupy many pages of this book, only a few of the most outstanding can be mentioned. Anaesthesia, introduced in Britain and America almost simultaneously in the 1840's, had made possible operations in surgery which no patient could otherwise have borne. Antisepsis, first used in the 1870's, and then asepsis, has banished wound infection as anaesthesia has abolished pain. Synthetic drugs, many of which have no counterpart in nature, now offer a wide range of new remedies for hitherto intractable diseases. Radioactivity and the X-rays—discoveries of the 1890's—can be applied to treatment. Hormone therapy, one of whose triumphs is the control of diabetes, has been developed. Chemotherapy sets out deliberately to manufacture new compounds for specific purposes. Beginning with salvarsan (1909) in syphilis, this branch has created, among many modern remedies, the potent range of 'sulpha drugs' which have defeated pneumonia, puerperal fever, and many another dread disease. From this has stemmed antibiosis, the combating of illness by means of naturally occurring substances having antibacterial action. Beginning with penicillin a whole new class of remedies has developed, and is still developing both in number and application. All this time too, the frontiers of surgery were widening; operations on the heart, the lungs, the eyes, the ear, the brain are now commonplace; scarcely an organ or structure in the body is now deemed inaccessible. Surgeons now have the aid not only of the few anaesthetics available to pioneers of the last century, but of new ones of undreamed-of efficacy as well as muscle-relaxants, heart-stimulants, anticoagulants, and haemostatics. In every civilized country of the world dedicated men and women are devoting hand and brain to medical research—a thousand of them for every one who laboured in this field only a few generations ago. The slow trickle of the stream of knowledge has become a rushing torrent.

We are now brought to consider the intention of such a book as this. It is not a sensational presentment of the romantic aspects of medicine, though the romance is there for a sympathetic eye to discern. It is not a history of the achievements of medical science, though these form its background. It is not a 'popular' medical encyclopaedia or even a domestic medical manual. No one will learn from it how to treat illness, though he will learn how illness is treated. It is not an elementary account of anatomy or physiology, though these topics have their place in its plan. It certainly is not a simplified treatise on pathology, but perhaps in intent it comes nearest to that definition. For its object is to explain the processes whereby the body becomes diseased, to make plain what is happening, how and why, so far as our present knowledge goes. Furthermore, when speaking of a disease which has yielded to the advance of science, some account is given of the 'rationale' of treatment. Where the cause of a disease is not yet known, our ignorance is frankly acknowledged—no speculations are offered, and the only theories mentioned are those sufficiently promising to be the subject for current research. Lastly, when there is no known remedy for a disease the book does not scruple to say so in plain terms.

In pursuance of this scheme I have selected a number of diseases which illustrate particular modes of causation, diagnosis, or treatment. Naturally, this selection has determined the inclusion of some diseases or the exclusion of others. Most readers will know of someone who suffers from a disease not to be found in the Index, and conversely some conditions which are there will not be familiar, and being unfamiliar may be deemed of less interest or importance. But if readers will patiently study the book as a whole, they will find its apparently disconnected sections do, in fact, fit together to compose a picture of the human organism in disease.

———

TUBERCULOSIS

TUBERCULOSIS means disease caused by the tubercle bacillus, and this can affect any part of the body. For example, tuberculosis can attack the bones and joints and the spine, and this 'surgical tuberculosis', as it is called, can be very serious. But here we will deal only with tuberculosis of the chest, or pulmonary tuberculosis—the 'consumption' of everyday speech.

Although many factors, including individual susceptibility, encourage the spread of the disease, its one essential cause is the tubercle bacillus—or, to give it its proper name, *Mycobacterium tuberculosis*. This is a minute organism, shaped, as 'bacillus' implies, like a short rod. (It would take some 8,000 average specimens, in single file, to span the breadth of a halfpenny.) Tubercle bacilli, which do not move about of their own accord, are very hardy and multiply very rapidly. Like other bacteria, they reproduce by fission: that is to say, an individual specimen divides into two separate offspring, and so on. This fission takes place about twice every hour—a simple calculation shows how many bacilli will spring from a single bacillus in the course of a day.

So much for bacillus; now where does the 'tubercle' part come in? Tubercles are little lumps, and the presence of these in the bodies of afflicted persons gave the disease its name long before the bacillus was discovered. Tubercles result from the entry of bacilli in this way: when the cells of the body try to deal with the invaders by surrounding them to prevent their spread, a mass accumulates (at first only just visible) consisting of both cells and bacilli. If the latter gain the upper hand, the tubercle grows larger. Nearby, other tubercles are growing in the same way. They run into one another and form bigger lumps called 'granulomas'. Soon the nourishment of the affected part begins to suffer, and the local blood-supply fails. The granulomas, now a formless mass, change into a different soft substance—a process known as 'caseation'. This is, in fact, the destruction of the normal tissue of the affected part (in this case the lung), and if it goes on, more and more of the lung is destroyed. The caseations 'break down' and leave holes where healthy tissue had been—this is termed 'cavitation'.

But the body does not easily give up the struggle. At all stages it puts up 'tissue defence reactions'. We have seen how, when they were first attacked by the bacillus, the local cells tried to arrest the spread of disease by 'walling-in' the invaders and if possible killing them. Failing in this, the body falls back upon other lines of defence. As the caseation process develops, the tissues surrounding the battlefield become fibrous; they form, as it were, 'scars' which attempt to put a boundary to the area of destruction. So the fight goes on—the bacilli striving to extend the processes of caseation and cavitation, the tissues trying to heal the wounds. Sometimes one side is gaining the mastery, sometimes the other. Sometimes the caseous mass, 'infiltrated' with lime poured into it by the surrounding tissues, becomes a harmless lump. Such calcified lumps cast 'shadows' in an X-ray photograph. Sometimes fibrous tissue encloses a cavity within a capsule. This imprisons the bacilli for the time being, but they are always liable to escape, and, when they do, they resume the attack.

It is easy to understand how serious a disease pulmonary tuberculosis is. The destruction of lung tissue means that a vital organ of the body has to work under a terrible and increasing handicap. This in turn affects all the other organs, for the lungs supply oxygen to the blood which nourishes the whole body. This accounts for the consumptive person's loss of weight and strength, and general decline. The distressing chronic cough, not surprising when we remember what is going on in the lungs, is an attempt to get rid of the material obstructing the breathing. The bleeding which sometimes accompanies the cough is from blood-vessels which, like the other tissues, have been broken into by the process described above. This disease, commonly fatal if untreated, kills at least 2 million people throughout the world every year.

The tubercle bacillus is found almost everywhere. It can live for a long time in a dried-up state, in a condition of suspended animation as it were. Then, if it finds its favourite environment of warmth, moisture, and nourishment, it 'comes to life', flourishing and increasing rapidly. As it is very common in dust, there is greater risk of infection in cities than in the open countryside. Some doctors believe that in crowded communities the bacillus is so rife that practically everybody is infected in infancy, through inhaling dust or air contaminated with bacilli: fortunately in the majority of cases the inherent powers of resistance prevent the development of the disease. If resistance is lowered however, through malnutrition or some weakening illness, tuberculosis gains ground. The disease is not inherited, but a tendency towards it may be, in the sense that persons who themselves lack resistance may transmit this deficiency to their children.

Means have been devised to detect the existence of the disease in an early stage, and even to discover a person's susceptibility to it. We have a large number of such methods, but the only one space allows me to mention is mass miniature radiography. This enables us to take X-ray photographs of the chests of a great many people in a short time. Although the photographs are very small (an ordinary radiograph is life-size) experts glancing quickly through them can pick out those which show signs of disease. 'M.M.R.' as it is called for short, is one of our most important weapons against pulmonary tuberculosis.

From what we have said about the body's attempts to defend itself against the disease, it is evident that anything we can do to 'build up' the strength of the tissues helps to increase their power of resistance. For this good food, fresh air, and rest are the first essentials and it was to secure them for tuberculous patients that sanatorium treatment was introduced. But they are just as necessary in the home as a safeguard against infection. Attempts have been made to 'immunize' persons against tuberculosis, analogous to vaccination for smallpox and inoculation for diphtheria; we have as yet nothing so certain as these, but a method called 'B.C.G.' vaccination is coming into use which many doctors think will ultimately be successful.

There is no medicine which by itself will cure tuberculosis. Those which are used are chiefly to relieve symptoms such as the cough. No 'disinfectant' is powerful enough to kill the tubercle bacillus without injuring the patient; but quite recently it has been discovered that an 'antibiotic' can deal with the bacillus without harming the tissues of the body. Antibiotics are obtained from various natural forms (moulds, fungi, and the like). They are able to prevent the growth of bacteria, but they do not act in the same way as antiseptics. Penicillin, the first antibiotic to be discovered, is still the best known. But the one used in tuberculosis is streptomycin. It is of particular interest because it can cure tuberculous meningitis, a disease invariably fatal before this antibiotic was introduced. Now, streptomycin is also used to treat pulmonary tuberculosis. Strange to say, its effect is greatly helped when the patient is also given an entirely different kind of medicine, a simple drug called para-amino-salicylic acid (a drug which is a distant relation of our old familiar aspirin and generally called by doctors 'P.A.S.'). Streptomycin and P.A.S. are each good treatments, but they are much more effective used together than either is by itself. Experiments are now going on with another compound called 'isoniazid', from which remarkable results are claimed.

When saying that rest is a necessary part of the treatment

of tuberculosis, we mean resting the whole body, avoiding undue exertion and fatigue. But there is a special local kind of resting. When we break a limb or sprain a joint, we rest it by putting it in a sling or a bandage in order to give nature a chance to heal the injured part. So it is with internal organs. If a lung is attacked by disease, it is logical to rest it so that its tissues can devote all their strength to fighting the invader. But how do we rest a lung, which normally we have to use all the time for breathing? There are several methods, all of which belong to a category called 'collapse therapy'; and all of which are based on the idea of putting a lung out of action temporarily while its injuries are healing. In the commonest operation of this kind, 'artificial pneumothorax', the wall of the chest is deliberately punctured and air is let in between it and the lung, the pressure on the lung causing it to 'go flat'. (We may think of these parts as being like a bicycle-tire, the chest-wall being the outer cover and the lung the inner-tube.) Sometimes when this method cannot be used, a more extensive operation called 'thoracoplasty' is tried—this involves cutting away portions of the ribs. There is also an entirely different procedure which depends on putting one side of the diaphragm (which plays an important part in respiration) out of action and consequently pushing up the lung from underneath, an operation which is termed 'phrenic crush'. The operation is performed on a nerve which controls the diaphragm; but the pushing up effect can be achieved in another way—by letting air into the abdomen beneath it, a procedure called 'pneumo-peritoneum'.

If nothing more can be done for a diseased lung, it has to be 'amputated', just like a limb too badly injured to recover. When only a portion has to be cut away, the operation is called 'lobectomy'; if the whole of the lung, 'pneumo-nectomy'. Such operations have become possible only within recent years, and even now they demand the highest surgical skill. But these extreme measures are, in fact, rarely called for, the methods of treatment previously described usually being satisfactory, so long as the disease is identified in the early stages. Indeed, increasing success is attending the treatment of pulmonary tuberculosis, and it may well be that, before many years have passed, the development of 'chemotherapeutic' measures will obviate the need for any form of surgery. Meanwhile, the principles of prevention and treatment discovered long ago are as sound as ever—food, rest, ventilation, sanitation.

NEW GROWTHS

WE are apt to take for granted many things which if we were not used to them we should deem miraculous. One such everyday phenomenon is growth. How is it that the various parts of our bodies grow to an apparently pre-determined extent and then stop of their own accord? How, indeed, do the different parts of our bodies come to be differentiated and complex? What happens, as you know, is that the human body comes into existence as the result of a union between two microscopic cells; these cells divide and subdivide, multiplying themselves until they form tissues, the tissues developing into structures from which all our organs grow. But how does this happen, how do these primitive cells (all precisely alike and few in number in the beginning) give rise to bones, skin, muscles, lungs, heart, digestive organs, the brain, &c.? We have not the least idea. It almost seems as if there exists beforehand an invisible blue-print of the individual, a mental picture such as an artist must have when he begins to paint or carve. Perhaps we shall never get closer than this to understanding the miracle of the continuity of life.

Some months after the first two cells joined together, the new living being is complete and ready to enter the world. You will note that it is complete, nothing is missing and nothing is superfluous. After birth, the individual spends a number of years in further growth—all very orderly and systematic—until he reaches maturity and stops growing. But all through his life every part of his body consists of cells (in countless millions), and these cells are now specialized in form according to the particular purposes they are designed for; nerve-cells differ from bone-cells, the cells of the skin are not like those of the muscles, and so on. But in spite of their diversity of form there is a general resemblance in their make-up, and they all reproduce themselves in the same way.

Cells are continually lost through wear-and-tear or injury, and are continually being replaced. The replacement is always exact—no more and no less than the proper number of cells is in existence at any time. This means that as long as we are in health our tissues and organs remain of approximately the same size and shape according to our age. That is what happens in the state of normal growth. But there are states of abnormal growth where something has gone wrong with the mechanism which maintains this precise equilibrium, so that cells begin to grow and tissues to proliferate without purpose—that is to say, the new growth is not necessary for any useful function of the organism, and is, indeed, injurious to it. These new growths may arise in any tissue of the body, any organ, or structure.

I have used the term 'new growths' deliberately, for that, simply, is what they are. But they are better known as 'tumours', and doctors divide them into two classes, innocent and malignant. The word 'tumour' means a swelling of any kind, and could be used of the temporary bump from a knock on the head, or the swollen joint of a 'tennis elbow', or sprained ankle. But, when a doctor speaks of a tumour, he usually means the permanent lump that results from the purposeless overgrowth of tissue in some part of the body.

Innocent or, as they are sometimes called, 'benign' tumours are not so void of ill effects as their names suggest. Their claim to these names is justifiable, not by reference to their own character but by the contrast between them and malignant tumours, which are much more dangerous. There are very important practical differences between these two, which we must now consider.

An innocent tumour grows and keeps on growing, usually slowly, and as it grows it presses upon its surroundings. This pressure may or may not be injurious, depending on where the tumour is. If it is pressing upon some vital organ it may seriously interfere with the latter's working. It may obstruct some important channel or impede some necessary movement, or the very weight of the growth may be an inconvenience, though nowadays it is seldom allowed to grow to a very large size. Though it may by pressure cause pain and danger, it is not of itself painful or dangerous to life, nor is it a disease which extends throughout the body. Usually such a tumour is enclosed within an envelope or capsule, much as a sausage is enveloped by its skin. It can, therefore, be removed easily by the surgeon, and once removed, does not recur.

Far otherwise is it with malignant tumours, generally called 'cancers'. Though doctors divide them into several categories, all are embraced under the heading 'malignant disease'. The great difference between these growths and the innocent ones is that the malignant tumour or cancer is of itself destructive to life. It is no longer a question of the mechanical pressure of a growth causing increasing inconvenience; the presence of a malignant growth, however small, is highly dangerous. As it has no capsule to contain it, it grows out among the cells of the surrounding tissues, destroying them as it invades. Small fragments of the growth become detached, and are carried away to other parts of the body, where they found colonies of malignant cells which in time expand into similar growths. Then the cycle is repeated. Thus a single, small, primary tumour, unless dealt with in time, may cause these secondary growths or 'metastases' throughout the whole body. As this malignant process can occur in any part, it may, by destroying the normal cells, attack a vital organ, and since a vital organ cannot be re-moved, the surgeon is powerless to help. Frequently, even when we think a malignant growth has been removed altogether, it recurs in the same place. And, of course, if secondary growths have already begun, the removal of the primary has no effect at all on them. Death, often within a few months, is the almost inevitable consequence of un-treated malignant disease, or cancer.

We do not know, though there are many theories, what actually causes new growths, either innocent or malignant. No doubt we should progress if we knew more about the mechanism of normal growth. Throughout the world, thou-sands of scientists are intensively investigating these prob-lems. The following facts have been established. Cancer can affect all living creatures—even plants—human beings of all races, primitive or advanced, savage or civilized, town or country dwelling. Its victims have usually attained maturity, it is uncommon in the young. It is not contagious, nor hereditary. It is on the increase—one form of cancer, that which affects the lung, has increased fifteenfold in a single generation, and is now causing nearly 10,000 deaths every year in Britain alone. (This rate of increase, the reason for which is unknown, is however exceptional, and some other forms of cancer are diminishing.)

Although we do not know the real cause of cancer, we

know that certain conditions predispose persons towards it. Such conditions seem to have one thing in common—continued irritation of the tissues which are ultimately to show malignant changes. This irritation may be brought about in innumerable ways; by mechanical or chemical irritants; by exposure to radiation; perhaps by the presence of viruses or other micro-organisms in the body; or perhaps because some old-standing local or general disease has weakened and irritated the tissues. Chimney-sweeps are liable to a form of skin cancer apparently initiated by contact with soot; cotton-spinners are similarly affected through lubricating oils; cancer of the bones has found victims among women who paint the dials of 'luminous' watches; cancer of the mouth has followed the friction of a pipe-stem or a broken tooth; workers with X-rays or radium, or with the materials of atomic energy, have been known to develop all kinds of cancers. It would be possible to go on for a long time with this list, but I must emphasize one very important point, that although these things appear to cause cancer and certainly have something to do with it, they are not (except, perhaps, in the case of radiation) its fundamental cause. Very many persons are exposed to these risks who do not get cancer, and many other persons have cancer who have never been thus exposed. There must, therefore, be two factors involved, something which renders the tissues liable to malignant changes, and something else which instigates the change. We know a good deal about the latter; of the former we know nothing.

Not infrequently the prevention, cure, or effective treatment of a disease precedes our knowledge of its cause. This happened, for example, with malaria, scurvy, and smallpox, and now with cancer. As yet we dare not say we can 'cure' cancer, but we can truly say that, taken in time, a great many malignant growths can be abolished or at least restrained. Such advances have been made in treatment that many thousands of people are living today who would not have survived under the forms of treatment known a few years ago. Modern surgery can deal effectually with any growth provided that it can be got at, that it is still 'localized', and that it has not irreparably injured some vital part. Either radium or X-rays can be used to destroy the cancer cells, while leaving the normal tissues unharmed. The latest development in this field is to employ 'radioactive isotopes', ordinary substances which are made temporarily to emit radiation just as radium does (they are products of the nuclear fission laboratories which have given us the atomic bomb). These 'isotopes' can be taken right into the body where they attack the malignant growth on its own territory. Having done their work they lose their radioactive properties and become simple molecules again. It may seem strange that radiation, which can cause cancer, can also destroy it; the reasons for this are too complex to go into here, but even in ordinary medicine we often have to use strong poisons.

Recently it was discovered that certain kinds of cancer can be treated by means of a synthetic hormone called 'stilboestrol'. Hormones are substances which the body produces for itself in certain glands and which have great influence on the working of our bodies (see p. 95). Stilboestrol, which is not at all like a natural hormone, but is much more powerful, is used to treat certain disorders in which the natural function fails. And now it has been learned that it can also cure some special forms of cancer, which is something no other drug or medicine of any kind has ever done before. But there are many forms of cancer which stilboestrol will not touch, and even with those which it does attack, if the patient stops taking the drug, the growth will recur. So we still cannot say that we have a complete cure for any form of cancer. One will assuredly be found some day to remove this scourge of mankind—the most baffling mystery of medical science—the malignant growth.

VENEREAL DISEASES

THERE is a group of highly contagious, very dangerous diseases which have in common one feature peculiar to themselves. In the overwhelming majority of cases they are caught and passed on only through the exercise of sexual functions. In this respect alone—the manner in which they are communicated—do venereal diseases differ from others. That is why they are termed 'venereal', which is another word for 'sexual'. They are caused by the invasion of the body by micro-organisms, members of the large class of minute parasites responsible for most infections. As all these organisms employ a similar mode of action in causing disease, all are combated on similar principles. It is necessary to make this quite clear before we go on—venereal diseases are not an inherent attribute of the sex function; but sexual union is the means of communicating infection if disease already exists in either of the participants.

The two diseases we have chiefly in mind when using the term 'venereal' are 'gonorrhoea' and 'syphilis', though there are certain others of less importance. Gonorrhoea and syphilis have nothing in common except their mode of transmission; they are quite distinct diseases and due to entirely different micro-organisms. Gonorrhoea is caused by a bacterial parasite known as the 'gonococcus' (or to give it its absolutely up-to-date name, *Neisseria gonorrhoeae*). It is usually found in pairs, and is rather like a haricot bean in shape with a diameter of about one-thousandth of a millimetre. The organism of syphilis is called *Treponema pallidum* (formerly known as *spirochaeta pallida*). This is not a bacterium, but belongs to the class known as 'protozoa'. It is spiral-shaped, rather like a thin corkscrew, and it is longer than the gonococcus, an average specimen measuring one-hundredth of a millimetre in length. Both organisms, like all similar agents of disease, multiply themselves with inconceivable rapidity.

In both gonorrhoea and syphilis the infecting organisms enter the body through intimate contact between the sex organs, but, as their effects differ considerably, it is convenient to study them separately. We will consider gonorrhoea first. Let us suppose that the gonococcus has passed from the body of the infected person to his or her partner. At first only the local parts are affected, and accordingly the symptoms are local. There is pain—sometimes very severe pain—in the act of urination, and there is a septic discharge. In time these symptoms subside, but this by no means indicates cure. On the contrary the disease, 'fanning out from the beachhead' so to speak, is gradually extending to the deeper parts of the body, unless a doctor has taken the matter in hand. It works its way upwards and causes inflammation of the 'urethra', the passage from the bladder by which the urine is voided, then inflammation in the bladder itself, and it need not stop there. The bladder communicates with the kidneys through two tubes called the 'ureters'; if the gonococcus makes a lodgement in the kidneys, the results are very grave indeed—they may be fatal.

There are further consequences of gonorrhoeal infection. Adjacent to the external sex organs are glands and other internal structures, to any of which the infection may spread. Among them are the 'testes' in the male and the 'ovaries' in the female—if these are attacked, the victim eventually becomes sterile, incapable of bearing or begetting children. In the female the interior of the abdomen is particularly accessible to infection from without, hence the very serious form of inflammation known as 'peritonitis' may arise. Abscesses may break out in the 'perineum' (the part of the body between the thighs just where they join the trunk), and these abscesses may cause 'fistulas', permanent openings on to the surface, through which urine drains—a most miserable condition. Blood disorders, certain forms of rheumatism and other affections of muscles and joints, injury to the heart or lungs, some kinds of eye diseases—all these and many other ills are possible consequences of gonorrhoea, unless medical treatment is sought. A very dreadful possibility is that a woman may have a baby whose eyes are infected at birth and who rapidly becomes blind.

Syphilis attacks in a different way. It also shows its first sign locally, but in the form of a small sore. There may be some local swelling, but as there is no discharge and no especially painful sensations, this early sign may escape notice. Thus left undisturbed, the micro-organism makes rapid progress. All sorts of vague illnesses and skin eruptions afflict the victim for perhaps years afterwards—in fact the symptoms possible during this stage of the disease are so varied that nothing is gained by listing them, for they may counterfeit those of almost any disorder. As a great physician of the last generation said, 'to know syphilis is to know all medicine'.

By this time the organism has spread throughout the body, destroying wherever it goes, unless medically checked. Ulcers may form in any organ and eat away the tissues around them, irreparably damaging the function of the organ. The ulcers may be in the skin, the muscles, the bones, the brain. Serious damage may be done to the heart and arteries, or to the nerves which control locomotion. Perhaps worst of all consequences is the condition known as 'general paralysis of the insane', which, as the name implies, is a combination of two terrible disasters. One very unusual feature of syphilis is that it can be in a manner inherited—in 'congenital syphilis', as it is called, the developing child is infected while it still lies within its mother's body; numbers of the *T. pallidum* which are harboured by the mother pass directly to the child by way of her blood with which the unborn infant is nourished.

The treatments of gonorrhoea and of syphilis followed quite different lines until recent years. No 'specific' medicinal treatment for gonorrhoea existed at one time, each symptom was treated locally, each various complication independently, as it arose; vaccines were also used, more or less satisfactorily. Then came the 'sulphonamides', which seemed very effective until it was found that certain disadvantages attended their use. For syphilis there was a sovereign remedy which, it is interesting to note, was the first chemical compound, not existing in nature, to be deliberately created for the purpose of killing a specific microorganism. This compound, originally called 'salvarsan' or '606' (it had later modifications as research advanced) was therefore the pioneer of the great branch of present-day medicine called 'chemotherapy'. Other forms of treatment were also used, alone or in combination with salvarsan compounds, with satisfactory results. But it still took a long time, perhaps even years, before a patient could be declared free from disease. By then, with both syphilis and gonorrhoea, lasting injury might already have been done.

The picture has been entirely changed quite lately. It has been found that both diseases can be treated effectively by a single remedy, the wonder-working antibiotic substance, penicillin. Other antibiotics too, are coming into use, and it seems that at last we have a means of destroying the infecting organisms wherever they may lurk in the body, in a much shorter time and with much less trouble to the patient than ever before. But it still holds good that the patient may not have been treated in time to stop some process that injures him for life. Treatment can be carried out only by experts, and self-treatment is out of the question; indeed, it is illegal for anyone but a qualified doctor to treat venereal disease.

Now we come to the matter of prevention, and here we are exceptionally fortunate. There are not many diseases which can be contracted in practically only one way, and that way easy of avoidance. It is true that there is a theoretical possibility of infection through contact with contaminated articles, but this is a very rare event, and the circumstances favouring it must be highly unusual. It may be taken as certain that practically every case of gonorrhoea or syphilis is the result of intimate contact with an infected person. Even 'congenital syphilis' is not an exception to this rule, as will be clear on reflection.

It is not to a book like this that anyone would look for moral guidance, or for a discussion of the ethics of sexual behaviour; nor are these offered here. But after writing technically of venereal diseases, I think it legitimate to point out that in illicit sexual relations there is a grave risk of infection, and that infection means at best undergoing a course of medical treatment, at worst, suffering a disabling illness. It is true that modern methods make treatment easier, cure more certain. But it is perfectly possible for the ordinary person not to notice the early symptoms of venereal disease, and therefore not to seek treatment. Although I have given above an account of the 'classical' course of these diseases, there are many deviations and delays in the development of symptoms. One may have become infected without exhibiting any of the signs described. And these observations are applicable to either sex partner.

PNEUMONIA

'CAPTAIN of the men of Death.' This quotation was applied by a celebrated physician to pneumonia, a disease which in his day and for long afterwards claimed its victims by the hundred thousand. Indeed, it is only within quite recent years, and as a result of a series of great medical discoveries, that pneumonia has been deprived of the grim rank Osler conferred on it.

Essentially, this disease is an inflammation of the lungs which 'consolidates' them, that is, converts their normally spongy tissue into a solid mass. There are two main forms, 'lobar pneumonia' and 'broncho-pneumonia'. The latter may be due to a variety of causes, the commonest being the invasion of the lungs by the germs of some disease already afflicting the patient. Diseases involving fever—which include several of the infectious diseases of childhood—can lead to broncho-pneumonia, as can any condition producing septic matter which may infect the bronchial passages. This is the kind of pneumonia which often arises in the course of a prolonged illness. There is, too, a kind which occurs simply because a patient has lain too long in a recumbent posture, the so-called 'hypostatic pneumonia'. Since broncho-pneumonia is usually secondary to some pre-existing morbid condition, treatment, recognizing that first things come first, tries to remedy this condition. The local infection may, however, have to be treated generally, in somewhat similar fashion to lobar pneumonia which we are about to consider. All forms of pneumonia still call for very careful nursing, notwithstanding the great advances in treatment.

Lobar pneumonia is a quite specific disease caused by a definite micro-organism, the 'pneumococcus'. It is a true infection, contracted similarly to other infectious diseases (see p. 28). After a short 'incubation period', it goes through a series of stages, as other acute fevers do. Its special features are the painful interference with breathing and other unmistakable indications of chest disorder. Its onset is sudden; the victim, probably after exposure to wet and cold, feels 'chilled', shivers violently, and may possibly vomit. His temperature rises to 103° or even higher, his heart-beat and breathing almost double their rate. He begins to cough frequently and to experience pain in his chest which increases to great severity. Actually, 'pleurisy' has set in. This condition (which can occur without pneumonia) is an inflammation of the 'pleura', the membrane which covers the outside of the lung. Pleurisy may develop into the graver condition called 'empyema', in which fluid exudes from the pleura and, being infected, forms quantities of pus in the chest; this has to be withdrawn by surgical drainage. Even if empyema does not set in, the pneumonia patient is very ill indeed. Formerly, the acute symptoms described above went on for a week or longer. If the victim survived for that time he reached a 'crisis', after which his symptoms subsided quite rapidly, though leaving him in a state of extreme weakness. An attack of pneumonia was generally considered to leave behind weaknesses that affected the patient for the rest of his life; and there is no doubt that he was rendered more vulnerable to many diseases of the respiratory system, and to certain forms of heart disease as well. The heart can be seriously, even fatally, affected during the course of an attack. The body, in a general toxaemic state as a result of pneumococcal infection, was liable to many morbid conditions, and the pneumococcus itself can cause meningitis (see p. 105).

Although pneumonia is caused by a specific organism, the pneumococcus, several distinct types of this organism have been detected. This fact was of practical importance

when the only direct means of treating pneumonia was by
the injection of a 'serum', for the serum had to be suited to
its own particular type of pneumococcus. It was not, however, always easy to determine the type of pneumococcus,
and in any case the serum treatment was much more effective with some types than with others. Nevertheless, the
serum method was the only specific remedy, the numerous
other treatments being directed only at the alleviation of
symptoms. During the 1930's the situation was so transformed that the 'typing' of pneumococcus has ceased to have
more than bacteriological interest.

This was due in the first place to the discovery of the
extraordinary antibacterial power of the synthetic compound 'sulphanilamide', a chemical used in the dyeing
industry for many years before its medicinal powers were
suspected. Next, a variant of this, 'sulphapyridine', was
found to be effective against all types of the pneumococcus.
Other 'chemotherapeutic' agents followed—'sulphathiazole',
'sulphadiazine', 'sulphamezathine'—till at last it could be
announced that the 'captain of the men of Death' had been
reduced to the ranks—though not quite discharged, perhaps,
for certain cases still did not yield to the new treatments.
But now came the antibiotics, the first among them penicillin, which either reinforced the action of the sulphonamides or dealt by itself with some cases which the
sulphonamides would not touch. Even yet there remained a
small proportion of cases of pneumonia unaffected by either
the sulphonamides or penicillin, singly or in combination.
It was finally discovered with surprise that these were not
due to a pneumococcus at all but to a virus. After this, they
did not baffle the doctors for long. First was tried, with
considerable success, another antibiotic named 'chloramphenicol' (chloromycetin); then an even more potent one,
'aureomycin'. Experiments are now going forward with a

still newer antibiotic, 'terramycin' which also seems highly efficacious. And so we add pneumonia to the growing list of the tamed tigers which for so long preyed upon mankind.

POLIOMYELITIS
(*INFANTILE PARALYSIS*)

THE popular name for this disease is 'infantile paralysis'— a quite inaccurate name, for it is by no means confined to infants and it does not necessarily leave the victim paralysed. The contraction 'polio' which is coming into use is a mean-ingless term, and there is really no satisfactory alternative to using the long scientific name. *Polio* means 'grey'; *myel* 'marrow' (i.e. the spinal cord); *itis* is the general suffix for 'inflammation'; therefore *poliomyelitis* signifies an inflam-mation of the grey matter of the spinal cord.

Poliomyelitis (to be exact, acute anterior poliomyelitis) is an infectious disease caused by a virus. We do not know the precise biological nature of viruses; though very much smaller than ordinary bacteria, they cause certain diseases in much the same way as these do; and in many other ways their behaviour resembles that of living organisms. Yet it is uncertain whether they can be regarded as being 'alive' in any ordinary sense of the word, so different are they from other forms of life—for example, some of them can be crystallized, and some are so small that they can comprise only a few molecules. These problems, however, do not concern our present purpose.

Among the viruses which cause disease some have a 'selective' action, that is, they prefer to attack only a certain kind of tissue. The poliomyelitis virus is one of those called 'neurotropic' because its preference is for the tissues of the nerves. It probably enters the body in most cases through the mouth, nose, and throat, a mode of entry used by the agents of many infectious diseases, both viral and bacterial. We believe that the infection is usually transmitted from one person to another by means of droplets of material discharged, for example, in coughing or sneezing. But there is another possibility with poliomyelitis, for the virus can be discharged from the body through the intestines. It has been found both in sewage and in house-flies, who are notoriously given to feeding on filth. It seems possible that the cycle may be something like this: a person carrying the poliomyelitis virus discharges it from the intestines, whence it gets into sewage; flies infesting this sewage pick up the virus and then, perhaps, convey it to our food; persons eating this contaminated food are liable to become infected. Obviously, water or milk could serve as vehicles for this particular mode of infection. A further complication is that some persons can be 'carriers' of the disease even though they themselves do not manifest symptoms.

The typical, though not the earliest, sign of poliomyelitis is muscular paralysis. What has happened is this. After invading the body in one or other of the ways described above, the virus spreads along the nerves until it reaches the spinal cord and perhaps the lower part of the brain—the part called the brain-stem. The region of the spinal cord most likely to be affected is the front part, hence the word 'anterior' in the scientific name of the disease. From the spinal cord proceed the nerves which convey to the muscles 'messages' from the brain to make a movement of any kind. When parts of the spinal cord are destroyed or injured, these 'messages' cannot be sent, so that the muscles do not act according to our will, the region of the body involved being, as we say, paralysed. There is a very serious form of poliomyelitis in which the paralysis extends to the muscles concerned with breathing. In old days this form was fatal; but now the patient can be saved by the application of the 'iron lung', an instrument which gives a continuous artificial respiration until the patient's own muscles can function again.

Although in many cases of poliomyelitis a rather extensive paralysis of the muscles and limbs sets in rapidly, a great deal of this passes off later. In some cases it disappears completely; but in most it leaves a part of the body affected, usually a limb. Unfortunately, when such a permanent paralysis occurs, it does not tend to improve at all. This is easy to understand: in those cases where improvement is possible, the spinal cord has not been injured beyond repair, so that its damaged cells may recover in course of time; but in cases of permanent paralysis the cells have been destroyed by the virus, and are no longer there to act as conductors of messages to the muscles. The possible success of any method of treatment, therefore, depends on the extent of damage to the spinal cord.

At present there is no known method of killing the virus in the body before it has done its work. We may be sure that some new discovery will falsify this statement some day, if not soon. Meanwhile, there is much preventative action which we can take about poliomyelitis. Knowing that the virus is conveyed by discharges from the body, we can secure that those discharges (whether they are from the nose, the throat, or the intestines) do not come into contact with any other person. It is not good manners to cough or sneeze at our friends anyway, and it may be dangerous. Although the disease is most prevalent in the summer, we can fight the house-fly at all times, paying particular attention to its breeding-places. We can keep our food and drink from contamination. When there are known cases of the disease in the neighbourhood, we can keep away from crowds, indoors and out-of-doors, and we can avoid swimming-pools. We should, whenever we are exposed to risk, avoid excessive physical exertion as it has been proved that a state of fatigue predisposes to infection.

If we are unlucky enough to become victims, there is still a great deal that can be done. At the beginning of the illness absolute rest in bed is essential. At the right time massage can be given, and then the limbs moved—at first, passively by someone else, then actively by the patient. Of all the people who get poliomyelitis only about one-half develop any degree of paralysis, and of these only a small proportion are permanently incapacitated.

SOME INFECTIOUS DISEASES

'INFECTIOUS' diseases include every disease which can be communicated from one human being to another, directly or indirectly. Obviously, it is impossible to apply the term so comprehensively in these pages. In other articles will be found accounts of various conditions, unquestionably infectious in the strict sense of the word; in this article I must confine myself to a group which have by convention come to be spoken of as 'infectious diseases' or sometimes (even less precisely) as 'fevers'. They are due to different agents, and they vary widely in their characteristics, but they have in common, though it is not exclusively theirs, the feature of definite 'incubation periods', that is, there is a certain lapse of time between the invasion of the body by the agent of infection and the outward manifestation of disease. The following is not a complete list of these diseases, but is a selection of those which chiefly affect the earlier years of life. As the incubation periods stated vary somewhat in individuals, I have generally given maximum durations. In some cases symptoms may appear somewhat earlier than the minimum figures—it all depends, as a famous lecturer might have said, on what we mean by symptoms.

Diphtheria (incubation period from 2 to 6 days)

This very dangerous disease, caused by a bacillus, used to kill 30 per cent. of its victims, who were mostly children. It first affects the throat, where the 'diphtheritic membrane' can be seen as a whitish patch. There is usually a raised temperature in the early stages, but in most cases this falls quickly, and throughout the rest of the illness the temperature may be below normal. There may be obstruction of the breathing passage—sometimes so bad as to cause suffocation were not an incision made in the throat ('tracheotomy' as the operation is called) to allow air to enter direct through the opening. Diphtheria can seriously injure many organs of the body, including the heart. It can lead to certain kinds of paralysis, including a generally fatal form affecting the muscles concerned with respiration. It is possible to ascertain individual susceptibility to diphtheria and also to confirm a doubtful diagnosis by the 'Schick test'. Immunization by means of antitoxin has reduced the formerly heavy death-rate from diphtheria to negligible proportions, and its general adoption would go far to abolish the disease. Antitoxin can also be used to treat patients who have actually contracted the disease, but obviously prevention is much better. Subsequent attacks of diphtheria are quite possible in those who survive a first attack but remain unimmunized, and 'carriers' (see p. 26) exist.

Measles (incubation period from 10 to 18 days)

The actual cause is a virus, but it is often complicated by a mixture of ordinary bacterial infections. The early symptoms are those of common catarrh. A little later small white spots ('Koplik's spots') appear inside the mouth. This is

followed by the 'rash', which is accompanied by fever, the
temperature rising to about 103° as the skin eruption develops. The feverish state lasts about a week. The rash
usually first appears behind the ears and on the forehead,
then spreads rapidly over the face, the body, and the limbs,
till in twenty-four hours it is everywhere. The complications
of measles are very serious, one of the gravest, broncho-
pneumonia, being often fatal. The ears are often affected
with an inflammation which may lead to total deafness;
sometimes the eyesight is injured permanently. It is not
easy to control the spread of infection owing to the long
incubation period, but it should be noted that the most
infectious stage is the earliest, when the catarrh causes
coughing and sneezing. There is no specific remedy for
measles itself, but the 'secondary infections' (to which the
complications are mainly due) can be treated effectively
with sulphonamides and antibiotics. 'Convalescent serum'
has been recommended for protection. A second attack of
measles is very rare.

German Measles (incubation period from 14 to 20 days)

This disease has nothing to do with measles, nor particularly with Germany. Probably caused by a specific virus, it
is rather less infectious than measles, though adults are more
liable to catch it. There is an early catarrhal stage and a
rash, both less marked than in measles, but there are no
'Koplik's spots'. There is, however, an enlargement of the
glands in the neck and elsewhere, a symptom not seen in
measles. The temperature does not usually rise above 100°.
As German measles is on the whole quite a mild disease—
it is never fatal, and second attacks are very rare—no special
treatment was considered to be called for, nor any extra-
ordinary preventive precautions. But it has recently been
discovered that if a woman contracts the disease in early

pregnancy her child is liable to be born with certain physical defects—and possibly, it is suggested, with some form of mental deficiency.

Mumps (incubation period 14 to 21 days)

A virus disease, easily diagnosed by the large facial swellings (they are really swollen 'parotid' glands) which appear near the end of the incubation period, and which usually affect one side of the face first. There may previously have been a feeling of unwellness, headache, perhaps ear-ache, sore throat, or 'chill'. The temperature does not often rise appreciably. Although mumps usually subsides fairly quickly, it can have some serious complications: in females the ovaries or the breasts may become inflamed, and in males the testicles; in very severe cases this can lead to sterility. There is no specific treatment for mumps; symptoms such as pain are treated individually.

Scarlet Fever (incubation period 2 to 4 days)

The cause is a bacterial organism of the class known as 'streptococci', but it is not quite certain whether one particular kind is to blame, or several. There are different forms of scarlet fever, some much more serious than others, and for many years the milder form has been most common in Britain. As in so many of these diseases, the first symptoms are in the mouth and throat, the rash quickly follows. The temperature may rise to 104°. A method called the 'Dick test' can be used to diagnose scarlet fever definitely, and also to test susceptibility to the disease, like the 'Schick test' in diphtheria. Infection is generally conveyed from one person to another through the secretions of the nose and throat, but healthy persons can harbour the streptococci and act as 'carriers'. In the more serious ₁orms of the disease various organs of the body may be affected, for example the kidneys may suffer from the inflammation called 'nephritis'. The joints may be affected by 'arthritis' (see p. 86). The ear may be severely affected, and 'mastoid disease' (see p. 124) may develop. An antitoxin has been prepared for the treatment of scarlet fever; antibiotics are also effective. It is possible but unusual to have a second attack of the disease.

Whooping-cough (incubation period 7 to 14 days)

This disease is caused by a definite bacillus, and infection is spread by 'droplets' from the throat of a victim, which need not be directly inhaled, but may be acquired from contaminated articles such as spoons and cups when only a short interval elapses between their use by an infected person and another. Again the early symptoms are those of catarrh, but soon a cough develops and turns into the familiar 'whoop', which is especially troublesome at night. There is only a slight rise of temperature, and no rash. Infectiousness probably diminishes with the development of the 'whoop'. Sometimes the whooping paroxysms are so severe that very young children fall into convulsions. Although the disease is not directly fatal, serious complications may ensue: the breaking of a blood-vessel, hernia (see p. 134), broncho-pneumonia, or the heart may be damaged by the strain of coughing. Injections of blood-serum taken from patients in the convalescent stage, and a vaccine prepared from the bacillus, are used both for prevention and treatment. A second attack of whooping-cough is exceedingly rare.

Chicken-pox (incubation period 12 to 24 days)

The cause is a virus, but chicken-pox has absolutely no connexion with smallpox. It has, however, some curious relation to shingles (see p. 136) which has not yet been fully explained. Before the appearance of the rash there are, in most cases of chicken-pox, only slight and indefinite signs of illness, rather more noticeable in adults than in children. The rash, which usually begins on the body and spreads to the limbs and face, consists of crops of small 'vesicles' rather like blisters, which afterwards form 'crusts' or scabs. There is not much fever, though the temperature may rise to 101° when the rash begins. Infection is spread not only direct from person to person but by means of mouth-contaminated objects and by shed scabs. Treatment is mostly confined to applications of antiseptics to the skin. A second attack is practically unknown.

Although these diseases differ so much in detail, there are certain general considerations which guide us in dealing with them all. First, nearly all begin with symptoms appearing in the nose and throat; there can be no doubt that many infections gain access to the body there—to put it in technical language, the naso-pharynx is a main portal of entry. Secondly, infected droplets of moisture ejected from the throat and nose frequently spread the infection. Therefore, any catarrhal condition in children which is not obviously due to a common cold should be regarded with suspicion, and precautions taken to protect others from droplet infection. Naturally, all recent 'contacts' with a known case of disease should be watched carefully until the incubation period is past. If symptoms of infection are manifested, isolation is practically essential. It is difficult to lay down a general rule for the duration of 'quarantine', which differs so much according to circumstances, but broadly speaking it is wise to keep the patient isolated at least until all active symptoms of disease have subsided. This may be excessively cautious in some cases, in others it falls short of what is desirable—compare whooping-cough and chicken-pox, above. In this, as in all things, the doctor's directions must be strictly followed.

THE SKIN AND SOME OF ITS DISEASES

MOST people regard the skin not as an organ of the body but just as an envelope or covering (the word 'integument' conveys that meaning) enclosing the body proper like a sausage-casing. But this is far from the truth. The skin is a highly complex organ which plays a vital part in the body's general working; if it is functioning imperfectly our health may be seriously affected. The familiar story of the boys whose naked bodies were gilded to enable them to take part in an ancient Roman pageant is an illustration of this: the impermeable coating of their skins is said to have caused their deaths within a few hours. The skin is made up of several layers which are traversed by innumerable blood-vessels, nerves, glands, &c. The 'pores', of which there are about 2,000 to every square inch, are really the mouths of the sweat-glands, part of the body's excretory system. The skin contains the 'end-receptors' of many important sensory perceptions. It transmits to the brain the sensations of heat and cold, pressure, and pain, it helps to regulate the temperature of the body. The unbroken skin acts as a most effective barrier against the entry of disease germs.

As might be expected of so complex a structure, the skin is liable to many disorders. A general disease of the body may extend to the skin, hence the outbreak of the 'rashes' of various fevers. Moreover, attack by many outside agencies can injure it. 'Dermatology', as it is called, forms a special branch of medicine. It is surprising that skin diseases are not much more prevalent, seeing how grossly the care of the skin is neglected.

It is impossible here to describe all the conditions which come under the notice of the dermatologist. Nor can we take as examples 'typical' skin diseases, for their causes and manifestations are so varied that the word has no significance. There are congenital conditions, nutritional disorders, and even nervous states which manifest themselves in more or less severe affections of the skin. Allergic states (see p. 149) often have a skin eruption as their only symptom. Various insect parasites invade the skin tissues, as do certain fungi. There are some tumours, both benign and malignant (see p. 11), which have a special predilection for the skin. A number of irritant substances, when brought into contact with the skin, attack it—the introduction of new chemicals in industry and even in the home has increased these 'dermatoses'. All these may be called the 'accountable' forms of skin disease, but there are many others of unknown or doubtful origin. Even the very common disease called 'psoriasis' is one of these, as are some varieties of the conditions vaguely termed 'eczema', 'pruritus', and 'dermatitis'. No useful purpose can be served by discussing these; we must confine ourselves to a few diseases where the cause is known and the treatment understood.

Scabies

This disease makes clear the distinction between the words 'contagion' and 'infection'. Scabies is strictly contagious, actual contact between individuals being almost essential for its propagation. Its outstanding feature is the intense itching it causes. From medieval times until recently a thriving trade was driven in alleged specifics for 'the itch' which apparently afflicted large numbers of people in the cities of Europe. Scabies was fairly common in Britain, but it was dying out under the influence of education in personal and domestic hygiene, and improved social conditions, until it had a revival just before and during the Second World War. It is caused by a minute parasite—a mite only about one-fiftieth of an inch in length and scarcely visible to the unaided eye, named *Sarcoptes scabiei*. This mite burrows into the top layer of the skin, travelling on the surface about an inch a minute, though when tunnelling beneath the skin less than half an inch a day. When the mite has excavated a horizontal burrow of convenient length it settles down to lay eggs, which it continues to do for several weeks—even as long as two months. As soon as the eggs hatch out—a matter of a few days—the larvae emerge from the burrows and wander over the surface of the skin while they are developing into adult mites.

Scabies causes an almost intolerable itching, especially at night. A rash, caused partly by the mite and partly by the patient's continual scratching, appears in the affected parts of the body. The scratching damages the skin and renders it liable to various germ infections. Some of these 'secondary infections' are of more than local importance because it is only the intact skin which protects the tissues beneath from the invasion of germs which may cause the body generally to be attacked by disease. But apart from this secondary risk, it is possible that constant scratching may cure the scabies, as the removal of the 'roof' of the burrows exposes the mites and may in time kill them off. This, however, is not a remedy to be recommended.

Scabies may be contracted by anyone—an attack pre-supposes contact with the mite and by no means lack of cleanliness. But such unhygienic habits as overcrowding, the sharing of beds, intimate personal contact, the mingling of school children with infected companions (whereby the parents, also, may become infected), and similar practices afford opportunities for the migration of the mite from one person to another.

Scabies can be completely and rapidly cured. Two sub-stances, sulphur in various forms and an organic chemical compound called benzyl benzoate, are particularly lethal to *Sarcoptes scabiei*. Benzyl benzoate is in more general use nowadays, because sulphur has a tendency to produce a dermatitis of its own, and also because it usually has to be applied in the form of an ointment which has to be rubbed into the skin over the whole body—rather a messy business. Benzyl benzoate, a non-greasy liquid, is simply painted over the body, and a single application usually kills off all the mites and their larvae.

Ringworm

This is a very different type of skin disease. Its technical name is *tinea*, qualified by a suffix to indicate the site of infection, e.g. *tinea tonsurans*, ringworm of the scalp. It has nothing to do with any kind of worm, but is caused by a fungus growing in the upper layer of the skin, in the hair-roots, or occasionally in the nails. Ringworm can occur in any area of the body's surface, but it is most common in the scalp and the part of the face where the beard grows—the latter variety, *tinea barbae*, is sometimes called 'barber's rash', though quite different conditions are also given that name. The ringworm fungus is visible only under a high-power microscope. There are in fact four varieties, the one most commonly concerned with scalp ringworm is *microsporon*, whereas that which generally affects the beard is *trichophyton*. The characteristic structure of such fungi is composed of a number of thread-like elements called the 'mycelium', and a vast aggregation of little globes called 'spores'.

The majority of cases of scalp ringworm occur in children. The disease is contracted from another child who already has it, but not necessarily by direct contact: articles such as caps, combs, or towels used communally can convey the fungus. It is possible also to pick it up from animals, and it is probably carried short distances by the air-currents in a room. The process of the disease is this: the mycelium of the fungus gets into the roots of the hairs, and as it grows it breaks up their substance, splitting each individual hair. When it has broken through to the surface of the hair-shaft, it forms masses of spores which envelop the hair; the latter, in consequence of its diseased state, breaks off at about the level of the scalp. It is now that the ordinary signs of ring-worm begin to be visible—the bald, scaly patches which give the disease its name. It is very infectious; it used to be not unusual for half the children in a schoolroom to contract ringworm within a month of one child's getting it. If un-treated, the victims may suffer for years.

The first essential of treatment is to get rid of the whole of the hair, not merely the diseased patches. There are several methods of doing this. A local inflammation of the skin may be deliberately induced by certain irritant applica-tions to make the hair fall out. Alternatively, a drug may be taken internally which has the same effect of 'epilation' as it is called. But the method in general use nowadays is to remove the hair by means of X-rays, a single treatment causing all the hair to fall out right from the roots in a few weeks. After a couple of months a fresh crop of hair begins to grow, and the scalp is now entirely free from the fungus. These treatments are applicable only to ringworm of the scalp and beard—when the disease affects other parts differ-ent methods must be adopted. It is quite possible for non-hairy regions of the body to be affected.

Impetigo

This is another form of skin disease, quite different from either scabies or ringworm. It is a true 'germ' infection, although no specific organism is known to be guilty. It is caused by members of the group of micro-organisms called *haemolytic streptococci* which are also responsible for many other diseases. 'Streptococcus' means a berry-like object which has a tendency to form chains (rather like a string of pearls), and 'haemolytic' implies a capacity for breaking up the red cells of the blood. In impetigo an organism of this kind gains entrance through some small abrasion, and proceeds to attack the tissues. It may be assisted by organisms of another kind called *staphylococci* because they tend to form clusters instead of chains. The first sign of impetigo is the outbreak of small blisters about the size of a pea, usually on the hands or face. These 'vesicles' are full of fluid which is crowded with germs. When they break the fluid runs out and dries on the skin, forming the 'crusts' which are characteristic of the disease. These sores, which exude germ-laden matter, make impetigo highly contagious, both through direct contact or via garments or towels. Impetigo chiefly affects young persons (though adults are not immune). In public schools it used to be commonly termed 'scrum-pox', football players often acquiring it through the contamination of their jerseys when hands or faces were rubbed against them.

Impetigo is not usually a serious disease nor of long duration. It used to run a course of from one to four weeks, but now that a penicillin treatment is used it rarely takes longer than a week to clear up. Penicillin is used either in the form of an ointment or a spray; the latter is probably more effective. It should be pointed out that if neglected, or wrongly treated, impetigo can pass from the acute stage into the chronic, when it becomes very troublesome indeed to deal with.

We can make no more than passing mention of some other skin conditions. 'Acne' is particularly a disorder of adolescence, occasioned partly by glandular disturbances but aggravated by faulty habits of diet, constipation, lack of proper exercise, and other factors (most of them well within our control), which lead to deficient blood-circulation and 'stagnation' of the skin. 'Seborrhoea', a more serious condition which, often first showing itself as 'dandruff' of the scalp, proceeds by way of 'greasy skin' until it may become the breeding-ground of many troublesome organisms including those causing a chronic form of dermatitis or inflammation of the skin. There is no specific remedy, but a healthy clean skin is not likely to be attacked. There are certain 'deep inflammatory dermatoses', as doctors call them, the classical skin diseases as the term is generally understood, which we cannot discuss here. There are two points which should be stressed strongly at the end of this article. Self-diagnosis of a skin condition is very unwise as there are many possibilities of error; and delay in obtaining effective treatment may convert a comparatively mild affection into an intractable one.

MALARIA

IF people were asked which disease is responsible for the greatest number of deaths and cases of chronic illness in the world, most of their replies would be wide of the mark. Heart disease, tuberculosis, cancer—these would be the probable guesses, with perhaps pneumonia, or some of the contagious diseases. These answers would be all wrong, for the greatest universal scourge of mankind is malaria, a fact which should teach us not to be too insular in our ideas.

It is a very ancient disease which, under various names, has been recorded from the earliest times, and which may be said to have influenced the course of imperial history. It occurs in almost all countries, attacking men, women, and children of all human races (there are indeed forms of malaria which affect certain animals and birds). Its ravages range from comparatively mild localized 'agues' afflicting individuals, to devastating epidemics killing thousands of victims over wide areas. But even this does not complete the tale—malaria is a recurring disease so that, although those afflicted by it may not indeed be sick unto death, at irregular intervals they are shaken by acute illness and incapacitated for days on end; the life of a sufferer from old-standing malaria can be wretched indeed.

In a typical attack the patient feels generally unwell, he has pains in the back and limbs, his head aches, he feels chilled. Then, suddenly, he gets much worse, he shivers from head to foot, feeling more and more chilled until he is shaking with intense cold. But in fact he is in a fever, so that soon he feels terribly hot, and a little later is sweating profusely. Then his symptoms subside, and he is left free from discomfort but exhausted in proportion to the severity of the attack. Many other features of illness are often present —vomiting, cough, &c.—varying in different individuals, but the general symptoms afflict all alike. From beginning to end an attack lasts for from five to twelve hours, and recurs regularly either every day or every second or third day, according to the type of malaria concerned (the explanation of this will be made clear later). When a person first has the disease these attacks may go on without slackening for weeks or even months. Then the intervals of freedom from attack gradually grow longer, but, if the disease is untreated, the attacks are liable to recur at any time, even years afterwards, and can persist throughout life. In some forms of malaria the symptoms are much more severe than those described, and the attack may run a rapid course resulting in death. There is a specially dangerous development, commonly known as 'blackwater fever', which is liable to affect persons who have already had a series of attacks of malaria.

Malaria is caused by a minute parasite, a micro-organism

belonging to the class called 'protozoa'. There are three, and possibly four, different varieties of the malarial parasite—all known by the general name 'Plasmodium'—and the type of illness they cause depends on which particular parasite is infecting the patient. Infection occurs through the bite of female mosquitoes of certain species of the genus *Anopheles*—only the females bite in order to suck blood from the victim. Many species of anopheline mosquitoes are constitutionally unsuitable for the transmission of the disease. These facts were discovered within the memory of living men, and how they were discovered makes an inspiring tale of heroic devotion and self-sacrifice.

It is over-simplifying merely to say that malarial infection is conveyed by a mosquito-bite. The mosquito itself must have become infected. How does this happen? Clearly, because the insect has previously sucked blood containing the plasmodia parasites from the body of a sufferer from malaria. But this is still only a very imperfect presentation of the cycle of events. Let us start with our original malaria-infected person. He is bitten by a female mosquito of the right species. His blood, containing great numbers of plasmodia, the malarial parasite, is sucked up through the mosquito's proboscis into its stomach. Within the stomach of the mosquito the parasites undergo a change of form and become capable of penetrating through the wall of the insect's stomach and escaping into the hollow cavities which constitutes the interior of the mosquito. They travel about until some of them get to the organs called the 'salivary glands' which are connected with the proboscis, the organ with which the mosquito pierces our skin and through which it sucks our blood. When the mosquito does this, some of its saliva containing malarial parasites is ejected—and injected. It is only by this method of 'inoculation' that malaria is communicated.

It is fascinating to trace the parasite through the extra-ordinary changes of form which compose its life-cycle. Per-haps the most remarkable feature is that the successive stages of illness in the patient—the preliminary symptoms, the cold, hot, and sweating stages—correspond with the varying stages of the parasite's development. For example, the cold phase is caused by the sudden release of numbers of parasites, which have been developing inside red blood corpuscles and which suddenly burst forth, destroying the corpuscles. There are about 5 million of these red corpuscles in every cubic millimetre of blood, and the amount of blood in the body averages one-thirteenth of the total body-weight (thus, a 13-stone man has about $1\frac{1}{2}$ gallons of blood in him). It is, therefore, easy to understand why such severe effects follow invasion by malarial parasites, even if only a small percentage of red blood corpuscles harbour them. When the parasite reaches a certain stage of maturity (and after it has made the patient ill), it cannot develop any more in the human body, but has to wait for a mosquito to suck up some of the victim's blood. Thereupon the parasite carries out further stages of its development within the body of the mosquito—then the insect bites someone else, and the cycle repeats itself.

Malaria cannot be passed directly from one person to another; no one can acquire it without being bitten by an infected mosquito. Our first line of defence, therefore, must be the destruction of the 'vector' (as such carriers of disease are called). We are helped in this by modern insecticides such as 'D.D.T.', which are sometimes sprayed from aircraft over areas infested with mosquitoes. Such methods kill fully grown insects, but may not deal effectively with them in their larval stage of growth. In this stage, the insect, as yet wing-less, lives in water, breathing through the surface-film. By covering the surface with oil, we prevent this manner of respiration, and the larvae die. This technique, combined with the draining of the marshy places where mosquitoes breed, has done much to eradicate vectors in many parts of the world. Where the risk still exists, protective clothing and 'mosquito boots' are worn, and finely woven gauze is used as 'mosquito netting' to cover in bedsteads and windows and keep the insects out. Then there are certain substances—a favourite is 'dimethylphthalate' or 'D.M.P.'—which, rubbed on the skin like ointment, repel all biting insects. There are odourless preparations, like vanishing cream, to be had, and these can be useful also for keeping off the British gnat.

But all these methods, though highly effective, are directed against the mosquito. How do we deal with the plasmodium, the malarial parasite itself? The most ancient remedy, and one still in extensive use, is quinine. The history of quinine is extremely interesting. It is obtained from the bark of the cinchona tree, and according to tradition, the Peruvian Indians treated themselves thus for malaria before the first Europeans reached America, and they later imparted the secret to Jesuit missionaries, through whom it became generally known. Quinine, which is an 'alkaloid', is the active principle of cinchona bark, and can be used both to prevent and to cure malaria. But as it is obtained from natural sources which might conceivably fail us, the search has gone on for at least a century to find substitutes of equal potency which can be made artificially. Within recent years success has crowned these efforts. Several synthetic compounds, in particular two called 'mepacrine' and 'paludrine', are now in common use—the first was known before the Second World War, the second was discovered in 1944. The war, by cutting off most of the sources of quinine, while at the same time greatly increasing the need for it among troops fighting in malarious regions, gave a strong impetus to research, and it is not too much to say that these new remedies made as great a contribution to the victory of the Western nations in some theatres of war as did almost any offensive weapon. Some lasting good has come to mankind even from those terrible years, for in certain respects the new remedies are superior to quinine.

All these drugs, including quinine, are designed to deal with the situation which arises when the victim has become infected with the parasite. This situation presents two problems: first, can we in any way prevent the bitten person from developing malaria; second, if he does become ill, can we cure him? The answer to both questions is yes. If the drugs mentioned above are taken regularly by people exposed to infection, the symptoms of illness do not appear. It should, however, be noted that in this case the drugs achieve suppression rather than prevention of the disease: the mosquito-bitten person with the malarial parasite in his body will not become ill so long as he continues to take the drug, but if he fails to do so, he will. The reason for this is that the drug arrests the development of the parasite's life-cycle at a stage earlier than that required to produce symptoms of illness. If, however, the illness has actually occurred through failure to take these 'suppressive' measures in advance, it can definitely be cured by administering the drugs according to special systems. As a final point of interest it may be noted that the efficacy of a particular drug is to some extent affected by which of the several varieties of the plasmodium is responsible for the infection.

TYPHUS

THIS deadly disease, now seldom known in Britain, but still a danger in some other countries, has absolutely no connexion with typhoid. It is unfortunate that the two names are so much alike, for these two different diseases are caused by quite dissimilar agencies. This article is concerned solely with typhus, in former times known as 'jail fever', 'ship fever', or 'camp fever', and so great a menace that prisoners in the dock brought out from a fever-infested prison were known to infect the whole court. Typhus causes high fever, outbreaks of blotches all over the body, delirium, exhaustion, and in very many cases death. It is associated with places where people are herded together under insanitary conditions. In the old days prisons, military encampments, and overcrowded sailing-ships were notoriously such places. That state of affairs has passed, but typhus remains a menace wherever dirt and crowded humanity exist together, and as these two things usually indicate a low standard of living, we may justly regard typhus as a disease of poverty.

A victim of typhus does not directly infect other people with the disease germs. They are conveyed by a 'vector', a living agent such as an insect, from one person to another. Let us first consider this germ, the true cause of the disease. It is not a bacillus nor a member of any other family of bacteria, and it is not a virus. It belongs to a class of organism we have not met hitherto in these pages, the class named 'rickettsias' after the scientist who first studied them. Rickettsias are very minute bodies, much smaller than bacteria. As with bacteria, not all of them are harmful, but those which cause disease act in much the same way as the larger organisms. The particular variety responsible for typhus is called, to give it its full name, *Rickettsia Prowazeki*, and its 'vector', or carrier, is the louse. We don't know how it gets into the louse in the first place, though some think it lives as a parasite inside its host just as certain worms live inside animals or human beings. We do know how the process continues. When infected lice get on to people's skins and cause irritation, the victim scratches the place, crushes the lice, and at the same time rubs the infection into the skin. Before long it has spread throughout his body and the rickettsia can be found in his blood. If other lice infest him they will suck up the rickettsia in the act of feeding, and if they get on to another person's skin the cycle repeats itself.

It will now be seen why close contact between persons is necessary for the spread of typhus. Lice do not move fast or far, and only lice convey the infection. Unfortunately, there are many parts of the world where the conditions favouring infestation by lice still exist. In eastern Europe and the Middle East typhus is prevalent, and in parts of Asia and Africa. During the Balkan wars which immediately preceded the First World War an epidemic broke out in the country then called Serbia (now part of Jugoslavia) and some volunteer British doctors and nurses bravely helped to combat it. During the Second World War it was feared that similar epidemics might break out in cities subjected to air attack, where thousands of the population sheltered nightly under very unhygienic conditions—in the London 'tube' stations, for example. Such precautions were taken, however, that these fears were not realized.

But a typhus epidemic did begin in Italy in 1943. When the Allied troops invaded Italy that country became a battleground and her chief cities were subjected to bombardment which utterly disorganized communal life and public services such as transport, water-supply, and sanitation. The conditions favouring the spread of disease came into being; and when typhus broke out it was apparent that immediate and drastic steps had to be taken. As ordinary typhus is carried only by lice, the obvious first line of defence is to destroy all lice. But the most powerful pre-war insecticides came from countries from which the war had cut us off— a grave disadvantage at a time when we had to deal with many disease-carrying insects such as the malaria mosquito. So chemists all over the allied world, from 1940 onwards, were seeking substitutes by examining a vast number of known substances to see if any of them would kill insects. One of the substances so examined was a compound called dichloro-diphenyl-trichloroethane (D.D.T.), which had actually been discovered seventy years earlier, but was not known to be an insecticide. In 1940 its powers were revealed—it was found to be much more lethal to insects than anything else available then or previously. No louse could live in the presence of D.D.T. But how to disinfest hundreds of thousands of people so quickly that typhus could not spread? This problem was solved simply by 'puffing' D.D.T. powder beneath the clothing with a little bellows—for thus great numbers of people could be dealt with very quickly by a small medical staff. So a typhus epidemic was for the first time in history stopped dead, and countless lives were saved.

One kind of typhus found in the Far East is carried by 'mites', and was responsible for much illness among our troops in Burma and elsewhere. Another North American kind is carried by 'ticks'. Mites and ticks are tiny creatures belonging to the same class of animals as spiders, and they can both be destroyed by D.D.T.

Nowadays we have a means of curing typhus when it has actually developed by the use of another member of the wonderful range of 'antibiotics' known as 'chloramphenicol'. Special interest attaches to it in that it is the first antibiotic to be synthesized—that is, it can be made artificially—an achievement which inspires great hopes of further developments.

SOME 'TROPICAL' DISEASES

THIS article is different from the others in that the widely differing conditions it discusses have in common only their especial prevalence in tropical and sub-tropical countries. Of the very many diseases called 'tropical', some are not strictly confined to such countries although they are most rife there. Two such diseases—malaria and typhus—have already been discussed. Most of the others I have had to exclude, but I shall consider in this article a few which for one reason or another are of particular interest.

Sleeping Sickness

This disease has absolutely no connexion with 'sleepy sickness' (*encephalitis lethargica*), the disease which, although we hear little of it nowadays, attained epidemic ('pandemic') force throughout the world some thirty years ago. Sleeping sickness, which is practically confined to the western and central parts of Africa, is caused by a microscopic protozoan organism known as a 'trypanosome'. (Other species of trypanosome are responsible for certain other diseases.) It is transmitted through the bite of the tsetse fly, rather as malaria is by mosquito-bites. Sleeping sickness, however, need not be conveyed direct by the insect from one human being to another, for animals such as antelopes can act as 'reservoirs' or intermediate 'hosts' of the trypanosomes. It afflicts its victims in various ways, the tendency to unnatural slumber (usually in the day-time) which gave it its name being only one of them. If untreated, the disease is generally fatal, and great numbers of African people have succumbed to it. Now that the cause and the manner of infection are understood, mortality is much reduced. Injections of certain synthetic drugs which mostly contain antimony or arsenic—

though one of the best is a compound of 'urea', a natural
by-product of the body—are effective for curing the disease.
It is possible, also, by the use of other drugs, to prevent
infection even in tsetse-ridden districts—compare the similar
use of drugs in malaria (see p. 40). Furthermore, large areas
have been cleared of the tsetse fly.

Yellow Fever

Lovers of old-time sea stories will be familiar with the
terrors of 'Yellow Jack', which once caused seamen and
soldiers to dread the prospect of being posted to certain
foreign stations, and which, in quite recent times, seriously
handicapped the construction of the Panama Canal. Nowadays it is practically confined to the tropical parts of Africa,
Central America, and certain regions of South America.
It is a 'virus' disease (see p. 25), and it is carried by a mosquito named *Aëdes aegypti*—not the same insect as the carrier
of malaria—which chiefly haunts the neighbourhood of
human dwellings. In the 'jungle' form of the disease it is
thought that monkeys may serve as 'reservoirs' or intermediate hosts. It is called 'Yellow Jack' because of its
victims' skin coloration. The disease affects the liver, causing
a condition of 'jaundice' in which bile escapes into the
blood-stream and causes a yellow tinge in the skin. Sometimes the condition is so extreme that the skin turns a deep
brown. It is a very grave disease, often causing the death of
its victims within a few days of their becoming infected, and
it is not unusual for one-third of all infected persons to die.
Unfortunately there is not as yet a specific cure, and all we
can do is to treat symptoms as they arise. The possibility of
prevention is more hopeful. First, of course, the mosquito
must be exterminated, and all houses where it harbours dis-
infested. Inoculation with 'serum' taken from a patient
convalescing from the disease confers some immunity, but

not for very long. Vaccination with a weakened preparation of the virus itself is believed to give protection for several years.

Plague

This was the 'Black Death' of the fourteenth century and the 'Great Plague' of the seventeenth. The former epidemic is said to have destroyed one-quarter of the population of Europe, the latter to have killed 70,000 persons in England. It exists to this day, chiefly in Asia and Africa. It is caused by a bacterial organism, the *Bacillus pestis* (sometimes called *Pasteurella pestis*) which infects rats with the disease. Fleas which have fed on the blood of plague-infected rats imbibe the bacilli and then inject them into the people they bite. There are several forms of plague, the commonest being the 'bubonic', so-called from the 'buboes', which are suppurating swellings occurring mostly in the groin though also in the armpit—and which were the first symptom the physicians of old looked for. A highly fatal disease, its death-rate in epidemics may be as much as 80 per cent. of those affected. Happily, it is easily controllable. As it begins in rats—the black or brown rats which usually come to England in ships —the first step is to kill the rats. The next step is to use powerful insecticides like D.D.T. to destroy the fleas. Preventive measures include special kinds of vaccination for persons travelling or residing in countries where plague is 'endemic'. For those who contract the disease there is now good hope of recovery by using sulphonamide drugs and the antibiotic streptomycin.

Cholera

This may fairly be described as a 'tropical' disease, for nowadays it is found chiefly in Eastern Asia; but only a few

generations ago it was a deadly menace to the people of
Britain—in one epidemic in England of less than a century
ago 50,000 people lost their lives. The germ of cholera, one
of the first to be discovered by the microscope seventy years
ago, is known as the 'comma bacillus' on account of its
shape, but is properly called *Vibrio cholerae*. Leading
symptoms of the disease are vomiting and a very severe and
persistent diarrhoea—the motions from the bowel are practically liquid. These two symptoms cause the patient to lose
body-water so rapidly that his tissues are dried up (de-
hydrated), a condition ultimately incompatible with life.
The disease is transmitted almost solely through contamination of domestic water-supplies by the discharges of cholera
victims. It is possible that in some cases it occurs through
similar contamination of food, and in this the house-fly can
play a part. It cannot be conveyed by mere physical contact:
as has neatly been said, 'cholera may be eaten or drunk, it
cannot be "caught"'. Cholera therefore is above all a
disease of insanitation; its disappearance in Britain coincided
with rising standards of public and private hygiene. But
sanitary improvements have not yet reached all the teeming
populations of the East, and there are still outbreaks of
cholera in which it is not unusual for 60 per cent. of the
untreated victims to die—many of them within a few hours
of being attacked. Apart from improved sanitation, the
isolation of infected persons, and the destruction of filth-
feeding house-flies, a special vaccine can be used by way of
prevention. Unfortunately there is no specific remedy for
those who fall victims. Treatment consists mainly of restor-
ing the lost fluid to the victim's tissues (in normal health
three-quarters of the body-weight consists of water) and of
relieving such symptoms as severe pain. Experiments are
proceeding with the injection of sulphonamides and antibiotics, and it is hoped these may bring good results.

Dysentery

This disease begins with inflammation of the bowel and develops into ulceration. It is characterized by severe diarrhoea (but of a kind unlike that of cholera), by passing of blood in the motions, and by pain and fever. But there are two kinds of dysentery, and although their symptoms are similar, they are due to totally different causes. One kind, 'bacillary' dysentery, occurs all over the world and is not truly a tropical disease, though it is commoner in tropical than non-tropical countries. The other kind, 'amoebic' dysentery, is definitely a tropical disease, being found mainly in parts of Asia, Africa, and South America. Unlike the bacillary form, which is due to an ordinary bacterial organism as the name implies, amoebic dysentery is caused by a protozoan parasite named *Entamoeba histolytica*, which is in many ways very like the common amoeba found in pond-water, although much smaller. At an early stage of its existence it is called a 'cyst', and the person who swallows these cysts becomes host to amoebae. They may be swallowed in water or food, or in raw vegetables or fruit that have been contaminated with the excrement of a dysentery patient, because of the local system of manuring or handling crops, or because of flies. A serious complication of amoebic dysentery is the development of an inflammation of the liver and the formation of a liver abscess, which is often fatal. The classic treatment is 'emetine', an 'alkaloid' obtained from ipecacuanha, though a number of new synthetic drugs are very effective. Antibiotics and sulphonamides are also used.

These are only a few examples of the diseases to which dwellers in tropical countries are prone. A number of such diseases are carried by insects. In the days of long sea voyages, none of these insects boarding a ship in a tropical port could survive until the ship reached a temperate country. But in the modern age of air travel a matter of hours, not weeks, separates us from countries where these diseases are 'endemic', and it is perfectly possible for disease-carrying insects to live long enough to transmit infection on arrival. This has actually happened—a devastating outbreak of malaria in Brazil some years ago was traced to African mosquitoes which had accidentally been carried across the Atlantic in aeroplanes. Very stringent precautions are now taken by all officials responsible for air traffic, for they are aware how easily and rapidly 'tropical' diseases could become universal.

THE ANAEMIAS

BLOOD is not a simple fluid. Rightly regarded it is one of the tissues of the body, differing from the rest only in that its cellular elements are widely separated and move about freely in the liquid medium which envelops them, instead of being packed closely together in the apparent continuity we are accustomed to suppose characteristic of tissues. The liquid component of blood is known as the 'plasma', and is itself of highly complex composition. It is actually an almost colourless fluid, the deep red hue of blood being due to the vast number of red corpuscles or 'erythrocytes' which are suspended in the plasma. These red corpuscles are disk-shaped objects only one-threethousandth of an inch in diameter; but it is estimated that the average human body contains 25 million million of them.

Mingled with the red corpuscles are the 'leucocytes' or white corpuscles, of which there are several varieties. Their total averages a mere 30,000 million; but they perform vitally important functions, particularly in helping the body to resist invasion by disease-germs. Other cells in the blood are the 'platelets' (about 2 million million of them) which play a great part in blood-clotting and in the repair of injuries to the tissues. Cells of all these kinds together make up the solid portion of blood—almost half its volume—but in this article we are concerned exclusively with the red corpuscles, and in speaking of these I shall make use of the abbreviation by which they are commonly known to doctors, 'r.b.c.'

The function of the r.b.c. is to carry oxygen to all the tissues of the body. Oxygen is essential for the maintenance of the processes whereby life is sustained, processes which are in effect forms of combustion. The blood, circulating generally through the body, gives up oxygen wherever needed; it returns to the heart via the pulmonary circulation where it is reoxygenated by the air breathed into the lungs. But it is not a simple gaseous form of oxygen which circulates in the blood—oxygen is taken from the air and 'fixed' by the r.b.c., that is to say, it enters into a very complex chemical combination with the substance of the corpuscle. The essential ingredient of this substance is iron, and the eventual product is a substance called 'haemoglobin'. This substance holds the oxygen until it is needed, and it is to the depleted haemoglobin molecule that fresh oxygen is restored through the pulmonary circulation.

There is a group of diseases caused by the failure of this mechanism at the most important point—that is, the blood is absorbing insufficient oxygen for the body's needs because the oxygen-carrying capacity of the r.b.c. is deficient. These diseases are known as 'anaemias', and a number of conditions are embraced in that category. However classified, they fall broadly into two varieties: the 'iron-deficiency' anaemias, in which there may or may not be a reduction in the total number of r.b.c.s, but in which, invariably, each corpuscle is short of its proper quota of iron (in the form of haemoglobin); and the 'dyshaemopoietic' anaemias, in which each individual corpuscle may have its proper iron quota, but where there are not enough r.b.c.s. Alternative names for the first class are 'hypochromic' or 'microcytic' anaemia (the one name because, being short of haemoglobin, the r.b.c.s are less red in coloration; the other because they tend also to be smaller than normal). The second class is also known as 'macrocytic' anaemia because the r.b.c.s are larger than normal although fewer in number. There are two other classes of anaemia of which I must make passing mention: the 'haemolytic', in which the r.b.c.s are disintegrated (see the article on malaria for an example of this), and the 'aplastic' in which the manufacture of r.b.c.s diminishes and finally ceases altogether through complete breakdown at the source.

It will readily be understood that anaemia is not necessarily a specific disease, but can be an accompaniment or a consequence of some other condition. It is obvious, for example, that rapid and severe bleeding can produce an anaemic state, as likewise can slow but prolonged bleeding. We have already noted one disease which affects the composition of the blood—there are others. But in this article we shall consider only those kinds of anaemia which arise, shall I say, spontaneously.

First, iron-deficiency anaemia. Now it is evident that haemoglobin cannot be produced in sufficient quantity if the daily intake of iron is insufficient; therefore we may expect this form of anaemia to follow serious errors of diet or hygiene. Until a generation or so ago every doctor saw a great many young girls suffering from what was termed 'chlorosis' or 'green sickness' (so called from the peculiar greenish pallor of the complexion); this was an iron-deficiency anaemia. It is practically unknown today, probably because girls have less restrictive clothing, more physical exercise, improved diet, &c. But iron-deficiency anaemia is still common among other groups of the community. It is treated quite logically by giving the patients iron in various medicinal compounds, and by giving certain vitamins which help the assimilation of iron, and hence stimulate haemoglobin production.

A very serious anaemic condition is 'megalocytic anaemia' (or pernicious anaemia as it is more generally known). To understand this we must know something about the way the r.b.c.s come into existence. They are made in the marrow of the bones—the red paste which fills the hollow cavities of the long bones of animals. Two things are essential to enable the bone-marrow to produce normal cells, and if either or both of them is lacking, pernicious anaemia follows. They are known respectively as the 'intrinsic' and 'extrinsic' factors. The first, which appears to be a secretion of the stomach lining, is sometimes called the gastric factor, while the second apparently has to be provided in our diet. But lack of these factors must not be confused with the deficiency noted in the preceding paragraph.

All anaemias are weakening to the victims, and consequently cause a general disturbance of bodily functions. But pernicious anaemia displays symptoms which are very much more striking, although sometimes slow to develop fully. Moreover, it is liable to give rise to a special and very serious complication called 'subacute combined degeneration of the spinal cord', in which there is widespread disturbance of the nervous system, perhaps going on to a form of paralysis. Pernicious anaemia was once a fatal disease, for which no treatment was of any avail—it was no use giving the patients iron as in ordinary anaemia, since they lacked the ability to utilize it in the production of r.b.c.s. But the picture has changed completely in recent years. It has been discovered that normal liver contains the chemical principle required to activate the bone-marrow to resume its function of producing red corpuscles. This principle, combining the intrinsic and extrinsic factors mentioned above, is known as the anti-anaemia or 'P.A.' factor. At first, patients had to eat large quantities of raw animal liver daily. This was unpleasant, but the alternative was to succumb to a mortal disease. Later on, it was found possible to make palatable liquid extracts of liver to be drunk. Later still, concentrated extracts were made which could be injected hypodermically in small quantities. Recently it has been found that the active principle is a vitamin known as 'B_{12}'. This can be obtained from sources which have nothing to do with liver, and when injected it has just the same effect as liver-extract. But the victim of pernicious anaemia, like the diabetic, has to go on with the injections throughout life.

Hitherto we have spoken only of anaemias which may be said to arise from 'internal' causes. But it is possible to produce anaemia—even a fatal form—by external agencies. These agencies include some poisons and drugs and certain industrial chemicals which, when absorbed into the body, reduce the number of r.b.c.s. Another interesting cause is radiation, that is, the bombardment of the tissues by X-rays or by the emissions of radioactive substances. These have to be used with great care, and doctors, nurses, and others who work continually with them have their blood tested frequently to check whether the number of r.b.c.s is falling below normal. New hazards of this kind have followed the discovery of nuclear fission, which is the release of energy through the splitting of the atom. The radiations which accompany this event are capable of inflicting very serious injuries on the human body, including anaemia of the highly fatal 'aplastic' variety. Workers in atomic research laboratories and atom pile establishments have to be safeguarded just as are the hospital staffs mentioned above. As may be inferred, the same consequences, but developing with a rapidity which defies treatment, attend the detonation of atomic weapons.

LEUKAEMIA

In the article on the anaemias we discussed the composition of the blood, and among its components the cells called 'erythrocytes' and 'leucocytes' were described (see p. 54). The diseases affecting the first have already been considered, but up to the present I have not spoken of a condition in which the leucocytes are concerned, the disorder whose name heads this article. Strictly speaking, I should have used the plural form as with the anaemias, but in leukaemia there is not quite the same clear-cut 'pathological' differentiation of the various types, so perhaps the singular is admissible.

Whereas anaemia is characterized by a decrease in the number of red cells, leukaemia entails an increase in the number of white blood corpuscles. It may be asked why this is to be regarded as a diseased state, seeing that the purpose of the leucocytes is benevolent and one presumably cannot have too much of a good thing. The answer is that the increase of white cells is really a manifestation of a morbid process akin to the purposeless overgrowth of tissues affected by tumours (see p. 11). We have already noted that blood may be regarded as a tissue: leukaemia may therefore be looked on as a kind of cancer of the blood, without involving local tumour-formation, nor necessarily running the rapid and grave course characteristic of malignant growths. The increase of white blood corpuscles is really an exaggeration of a natural phenomenon; for a physiological increase also takes place if the body is invaded by disease germs when the leucocytes are, so to speak, mobilized in strength to repel the attack. There are, too, diseases characterized by a decrease in the number of leucocytes—analogous to the r.b.c. (red blood corpuscle) deficiency of anaemia; but we shall not discuss these here.

Leucocytes are manufactured chiefly by the 'spleen' and in the 'lymphatic glands', though there are other sources, including the bone-marrow already encountered in connexion with r.b.c.s. The spleen is a distinct organ, lying in the abdomen on the left side of the upper region. There are many lymphatic glands scattered throughout the body, forming part of the 'lymphatic system', one of the vital systems of the body, as important in its way as is the circulation of the blood. 'Lymph', a fluid derived from the blood by permeation through the walls of capillaries (see p. 67), bathes all tissues. This fluid, like the blood, is circulated throughout the body by means of special vessels, and at intervals along the course of these vessels are situated the lymphatic glands. They have several important functions, but the one with which we are immediately concerned is their connexion with the manufacture of leucocytes.

In leukaemia there is invariably an overgrowth of the tissues responsible for producing leucocytes, resulting inevitably in over-production. Like anaemia, leukaemia may roughly be divided into two separate categories, but the classification is based on quite different principles. What determines the category of the leukaemia is whether the organs primarily affected are the lymph-glands or the other 'manufactories'. If the first, the condition is termed 'lymphatic leukaemia'; if the second, 'myeloid leukaemia'. Both types are chronic diseases in that, although they are fatal, the sufferer may live for some years. But there is an acute form in which all organs responsible for leucocyte-production are affected, and which is therefore both myeloid and lymphatic. This form runs a very rapid course, and death ensues in a matter of weeks, or months at the most. It is noteworthy that although at first leukaemia's most remarkable feature is the great increase in the number of leucocytes, later the erythrocytes claim attention, for during the course of the disease there develops an anaemia which may be one of either of the types described on p. 55. Thus in time both of the principal cellular elements of the blood are affected, and sometimes one can literally use the graphic phrase: 'His blood turned to water.'

The commonest form of leukaemia is the myeloid, in which the most marked symptom is the enlargement of the spleen. This is not peculiar to leukaemia, for it can occur in other diseases, yet here the overgrowth is very great. The patient becomes weak, and loses flesh—although dropsical from accumulations of fluid—and dies eventually from general exhaustion. In the lymphatic form also the spleen enlarges, but in addition there is swelling both of the lymph-glands throughout the body, and of the liver. The patient nevertheless loses weight, and dies either from sheer weakness, or more usually from some 'intercurrent' diseased state, for example, an infection which the body no longer has the power to resist. Acute leukaemia accelerates all the symptoms described above, and has some special mani-festations of its own, including ulceration, tumours of various parts of the body (including the bones), and bleeding into the tissues—particularly the skin, which quickly develops the dark spots or patches called 'purpura'. All kinds of leukaemia are commoner in males than females; the lymphatic variety does not often occur before late middle age, the myeloid somewhat earlier; the acute form affects mostly children and youths.

The only means of treatment which are at all effectual

(and they only prolong life in the chronic varieties of the disease) are those which prevent the increased production of leucocytes. It should here be remarked that a great number of these excess cells are not fully grown white blood corpuscles, but are 'immature' or 'primitive'. To destroy them at this early stage is the aim of all the various forms of treatment. The great stand-by is 'X-ray therapy', but experimental work is going on with the 'radioactive isotopes' mentioned on p. 16—in this case the element used is phosphorus. There are also certain drugs of value because they inhibit the growth of the unwanted cells. One such drug, called 'urethane', is taken by the mouth. Another, the oddly named 'nitrogen-mustard' (a variant of the blistering gas used in the First World War, dichloro-diethyl-sulphide, with a nitrogen molecule substituted for sulphur) must be injected into the veins, and directly reduces the number of leucocytes. The general opinion among doctors is that X-rays are still the most efficient means we have of alleviating the very serious disease leukaemia in all its forms—unhappily, we cannot yet say, of 'curing' it.

THROMBOSIS

LATER on in this book (see p. 142) we shall consider the importance of blood-clotting, the coagulative property of the blood essential to life and health. But it is possible to have too much of a good thing, and we shall now consider the effects of coagulation in the wrong place, that is, 'thrombosis' (*thrombus* = a clot).

Normally, blood clots only when it is shed, and then only at the site of the injury. But by a slightly different process in certain states of ill health clots form inside the body's living blood-vessels, the arteries or the veins. It is easy to see that this can lead to serious consequences, according to the situation of the clot. For example, a clot of blood which blocks an important vessel such as the coronary artery (one of the arteries which serve the heart) can cause either instant death or very severe and prolonged illness; a clot in one of the vessels of the brain can cause paralysis. The first of these conditions is known as 'coronary thrombosis', the second 'cerebral thrombosis'. Even in a small vessel a clot can have dire results, for example, the blocking of the retinal artery causes sudden and permanent loss of sight. It is possible for a clot to form inside the heart itself. Happily, most occurrences of thrombosis are not in these vital regions: but, wherever it occurs, it gives rise to disagreeable symptoms.

Let us see how it comes about. Broadly speaking, anything which slows down the movement of the blood circulating through the body tends to produce thrombosis through a kind of local stagnation. Slowing-down can be brought about in several ways, and one of these is the general enfeeblement caused by old age or illness. Any condition which causes the normally smooth lining of the blood-vessels to become rough also checks the current and favours coagulation of the blood. A main exciting cause of thrombosis is inflammation of the veins, the condition called 'phlebitis'. This condition is generally due to various germ infections, but sometimes to certain poisons in the blood, and sometimes to local injuries which do not actually cause the wall of a vessel to be broken.

When once a clot forms, it usually sticks to the lining of the vein or artery. It may be big enough to fill the 'bore' completely, fitting like a plug and preventing any blood from getting past it, so that all the parts beyond suffer from being deprived of blood-supply. This deprivation may have serious results. These results are not always immediate as the blood will usually find another way round, like traffic in a blocked main road. A clot which does not block the vessel may, if it becomes detached from the lining of the vein or artery, be an even greater potential danger. It may be carried away with the blood-stream and then stick in some other part of the body where it may cause more serious damage. A loose clot which obstructs a blood-vessel is called an 'embolus'.

There is an interesting kind of thrombosis associated with a condition known as *thrombo-angiitis obliterans*, or 'Buerger's Disease', of which the late King George VI was a sufferer. It begins with an inflammation of the blood-vessels, as in phlebitis. We do not know the cause of the inflammation in Buerger's Disease, but it may be an infection. Whatever the cause, the result is thrombosis—not a single clot, however, but a widespread condition affecting a number of vessels, in the legs and arms chiefly, but especially the legs. The thrombosis is of the 'occlusive' or plugging-up variety mentioned in the preceding paragraph, the kind that completely blocks the vessels and shuts off the circulation. The sufferer, who usually has a good deal of pain in the feet and legs, gradually becomes unable to walk. In advanced cases there is ulceration of the affected parts and perhaps even gangrene which necessitates amputation.

At one time medical opinion was divided on the treatment of thrombosis. One school of thought advocated detaching and breaking up the clot, while another, fearing the danger of wandering clots or emboli, strove to attach it more firmly where it was. In some desperate cases an attempt was made to cut out the piece of the vein or artery where the clot had lodged, but this was not often possible. Nowadays a main line of treatment is rest, for it is recognized that the essential feature of thrombosis is the inflammation of the blood-vessels, and the inflammation is more likely to subside if the least possible strain is put on the blood-vessels. There has of late been an interesting development, however, which promises more direct results. As I have said, the danger in breaking up the clot is that portions of it may float away in the blood and lodge somewhere to cause even more serious trouble. Obviously, if a method could be devised whereby the clot could be gently dissolved away, this risk would not exist. Such a method is found in 'anti-coagulant therapy'. Anticoagulants are substances which prevent blood from clotting; a typical example, 'heparin', occurs naturally in some organs of the body, but other substances with like properties can be made artifically. When there is reason to fear the formation of thrombi—for instance in patients who have undergone certain surgical operations—they are given anticoagulants which, by keeping their blood liquid, avert this peril. Heparin is also used to treat thrombosis where it has actually occurred, and a curious feature during this treatment is that the patient is encouraged to move about, instead of submitting himself to absolute rest. 'Sympathectomy' (see p. 72) is sometimes performed. Of course, these special methods are not suitable for every case, and they must be applied only under the strictest medical supervision. I began this article by saying that it is possible to have too much of a good thing (meaning then, blood-clotting), and I end with the reminder that the other extreme—undue fluidity of the blood—is equally undesirable!

VARICOSE VEINS

PREVALENT fashions, including that of going stockingless in summer, disclose physical defects which might otherwise have remained concealed. In particular, we notice that many people, men of course as well as women, have very prominent veins in their legs, dark blue in colour and sometimes showing knots or bunches along their length. These are 'varicose' veins. The word 'varicose' is derived from *varus* = 'crooked', which exactly describes the appearance of the veins on the surface.

Varicose veins not only look, but are, unpleasant. They are most common in the legs, but veins in any part of the body can become varicose. Even the little veins in the lining of the stomach, the throat, and nose, and other organs sometimes get into this swollen and stretched condition. One special kind of varicose vein results in 'haemorrhoids' or 'piles'—swellings of the veins in the lower rectum (the section of the large intestine terminating at the anus). With males a similar type of varicose vein, called 'varicocele', may appear in the testicle.

All varicose conditions are uncomfortable, painful, or even dangerous. Varicose veins in the legs cause aching and tiredness, especially during long periods of standing, and sometimes quite severe pain. Haemorrhoids make bowel emptying difficult and painful, and cause much local irritation. Small varicose veins in the internal organs may break, giving rise to serious haemorrhage. External veins, such as those in the leg, may also burst or be punctured and thus cause loss of large quantities of blood. There are many minor disorders associated with varicose veins, one being a form of eczema, and another ulceration.

What, then, causes veins to become varicose? It is believed that an hereditary tendency exists in the first place, but that the immediate cause is a degeneration in the walls of the veins. The circulatory system includes two quite different kinds of blood-vessels, veins and arteries. Arteries, tubes of various diameters which convey to the tissues the blood the heart is continually pumping out, have walls of several layers (like certain kinds of hose-pipe), and this enables them to combine muscular action with elasticity so as to regulate the flow of blood through them. The 'bore' of a healthy artery is perfectly smooth and structureless, for it must oppose no obstruction to the stream. But veins, which exist to return the blood to the lungs, although outwardly resembling arteries, are differently constructed internally. Spaced out at intervals along their 'bore' are a series of valves whose function—much like that of the non-return valves familiar in mechanics—is to prevent blood flowing in the wrong direction. These valves look rather like small waistcoat pockets attached to the inside wall of the vein. They all have their openings (the mouths of the pockets) placed so that blood flows readily past them in one direction only, for, if it tries to flow back, the pockets open out and spread across the bore of the vein to stop the back-flow. The principle is like that of the valve of a cycle-tire which lets air in but not out.

It may seem strange that the arteries need no such safeguard against back-flow. If the artery–vein system were directly connected, they would; but there is no such direct connexion. There is indeed a flow-and-return system of circulation of the blood throughout the body, but it is not like a plumber's 'closed circuit'. When an artery has run its course it is not immediately connected to a vein. The blood it carries passes through a series of branching channels of diminishing diameter into a fine network of exceedingly small vessels called 'capillaries'. On the other side of this capillary network the veins take on their job of returning the 'used' blood to the heart. We can now understand why veins require valves and arteries do not. In the arteries the blood flows under the impulsion of the heart-beat, with a 'positive thrust' behind it. In the veins this force is lacking. Moreover, many veins are subject to some outside pressure (for example, from the movements of adjacent muscles) which tends to make the blood flow backward until checked by the valves.

It is easy to see why veins are prone to varicosity. Loss of elasticity in their walls (which anyway are much thinner than those of arteries) dilates them permanently, and the valves, by holding up the continuous flow of blood, create stagnant pools. And so we get our stretched, swollen, crooked, knotty, 'varicose' veins with all their attendant discomforts. But what can we do for them? If they are in the commonest place, the legs, the relaxed veins can be supported artificially, generally by means of elastic bandages or stockings, which give great relief, but of course do not effect a cure. If the condition is very bad so that the patient can scarcely get about, no amount of bandaging is of much service. In such severe cases the only remedy until recent years was a surgical operation in which the varicose vein was cut out of the circulation; the blood which used to flow through it will in that case find another way round.

A method is now very commonly employed which does not call for surgery in the strict sense of the word. The same object, to block up the vein concerned, is achieved differently. A certain chemical solution is injected into the vein which causes a mild inflammation of its wall. (This carefully controlled inflammation must not be confused with the serious condition 'phlebitis'.) This provokes a local reaction in the form of a blood-clot—ordinarily a very undesirable thing to have in a vein, but this deliberately induced blood-clot soon turns into a very tough plug which cannot move about to cause 'embolism' (see p. 64). This has the same effect as the surgical operation described above, a permanent cure of the varicosity.

Haemorrhoids are also treated successfully by this method, which has the great advantage that the patient is not as a rule laid up. The injection method is not, however, suitable for the treatment of varicocele, or of those varicose veins of the internal organs mentioned earlier.

HYPERTENSION
(*HIGH BLOOD-PRESSURE*)

ADMIRERS of *Little Dorrit* will remember that until the truth came out about Mr. Merdle, his end was popularly attributed to 'pressure'. From the text we infer that this term was meant to indicate some mysterious weight on his brain, whereas in fact his only burden was that of his sins. Nowadays very little is heard publicly about either of these forms of pressure, but we do very commonly hear of another kind. Almost everybody knows someone of whom it is said: 'He has blood-pressure', and I propose to say something about this oddly inaccurate term.

Blood-pressure itself is not a disease; indeed, it is a physiological quality without which we could not live. If we think of the circulatory system as though it were an ordinary piece of plumbing, a powerful pump might be said to be forcing a continuous supply of liquid through a series of pipes, some of which are above its own level. The pump has to carry on its work no matter what the gravitational or environmental conditions. Under the thrust of the heart's pulsations the blood is driven through the arteries, overcoming a considerable resistance as it is impelled on its journey. In these circumstances it is obvious that the blood must be under pressure; if the pressure failed, the circulation would cease. To use the term 'blood-pressure' to denote disease is therefore absurd. What it is intended to convey is that the pressure of blood is abnormally high. There is a condition too, in which it is abnormally low, but as this is much less common we shall not discuss it here. We shall confine ourselves to describing high blood-pressure, technically called 'hypertension'.

If we feel the pulse in the wrist, we perceive a rhythmic throbbing which represents a remote consequence of the heart-beat, and we can easily detect with each beat that the blood is definitely under pressure. If an artery is cut, the blood does not gush out in a continuous stream but spurts forth in jets corresponding with the heart-beats; here again we have a plain demonstration of pressure. It is indeed possible to detect the variation of pressure between 'systole' (the phase of contraction of the heart when it is driving blood out) and 'diastole' (the phase of expansion or, we might say, relaxation, when it is taking blood in). We can also measure these pressures by means of an instrument called the 'sphygmomanometer'. A healthy man in the prime of life has a 'systolic pressure' sufficient to raise a column of mercury to a height of about 150 millimetres, sinking to about 90 millimetres in diastole. As these figures can vary quite considerably in individuals without indicating disease, they must be taken only as averages.

But there is a condition in which the blood-pressure readings are consistently higher than average, even allowing for these normal variations. This condition, 'essential hypertension', is definitely a disease, although not necessarily a serious one. Persons, mostly men, who have reached middle age are most liable to it, and many are so affected. The symptoms, apart from the raised blood-pressure, are very varied. They develop gradually, at first causing no more than slight discomfort—headache, noises in the ears, perhaps a little palpitation, giddiness, and liability to fatigue. If the disease progresses, more important symptoms arise because the heart and the arteries, and probably the kidneys, may become impaired. A condition in which the pressure inside the blood-vessels is always higher than it should be imposes strains upon them which must in time have a bad effect. The heart enlarges, the walls of arteries harden, there may be internal bleeding in certain organs (including the eye), the function of the bladder may be disturbed. After perhaps many years, the patient dies of heart failure or cerebral haemorrhage (bleeding into the brain caused by the breaking of some small vessels in that region). There is an acute form of the condition termed 'malignant hypertension'. In this, the symptoms are much more severe and the course much more rapid. The blood-pressure is higher than in the 'essential' form (which is sometimes called 'benign' by way of distinction) and early death is inevitable —a victim of malignant hypertension rarely lives more than two years after the onset of this disease.

There is no lack of theories to account for hypertension; few medical topics have had so much ink spilt over them. The immediate cause of the raised pressure is that the 'bore' of the arteries is too small for the volume of blood flowing through them. It can be shown by a simple experiment with a tank full of water and outflow pipes of different diameters that the smaller the bore, the greater the pressure. But hypertensive patients do not as a rule start out with oversized hearts and rigid arteries—they get that way as the disease advances. What is it that instigates the process? One possibility is that it begins with some abnormality of the kidneys, which are highly complex organs intimately associated with the circulation of the blood. The kidneys regulate the composition of the blood in certain vital respects, and every drop of blood in the body has to pass through them in the course of its journey. If they are damaged, it is easy to see that a kind of 'back-pressure' may be set up through the obstruction of the blood-flow. It is possible that kidney disease, and perhaps some disorders of the 'endocrine system' (see p. 95), may produce a substance capable of directly constricting blood-vessels and thereby raising their internal pressure. Another possibility is that the normal metabolism of the body is deranged by an excess of nitrogenous foods—proteins—causing tissue-changes. But it is profitless to pursue here the numerous theories of the causation of hypertension, all of which have their advocates among medical scientists. Quite probably there is no single cause—many different conditions may, alone or in combination, be responsible for the symptoms in different individuals.

As we do not know the cause of essential hypertension, its treatment must be to some extent empirical; but we do know enough of its nature to deduce some conclusions about its treatment. Since this is another disease the course of which is powerfully influenced by the state of the patient's mind, intense mental concentration, violent emotion, prolonged anxiety, undue excitement—all these must be avoided in this as in most forms of cardio-vascular disease. John Hunter spoke very truly in the eighteenth century when he said that his life was at the mercy of 'any scoundrel who chose to annoy him'. There are many restraints on the physical activities of the hypertensive patient, too, but the modern practice is not to constrict normal life more than necessary. Tranquillity of mind is more important, and this generally calls for the regular use of some kind of sedative drug. It is doubtful whether any drug directly benefits the rising blood-pressure—those which depress it have drawbacks of their own. But some which have recently been experimented with promise better results. An extremely interesting development is the application of surgery to hypertension. It has been found that appreciable benefit sometimes follows an operation on the 'sympathetic (autonomic) nervous system'. It is impossible to give a simple explanation of this; but it may be said briefly that the sympathetic nervous system is concerned, *inter alia*, with regulating the elasticity of the walls of blood-vessels; if we divide the nerves which supply arteries, the arteries are allowed to dilate more than usual, and the increase of 'bore' relieves the internal pressure. This operation of 'sympathectomy' has been successfully practised in relieving other conditions; its use in hypertension is still in the pioneer stage.

ANGINA PECTORIS

'HEART DISEASE' has been nearly as useful as a 'decline' to the nineteenth-century novelist who wished to excite sympathy for a situation or to kill off an inconvenient character. The 'heart disease' of the novel was usually of sudden onset and swiftly fatal. In fact, however, there are not many forms of cardiovascular illness which correspond at all closely to the novelist's idea; but there is one of particularly dramatic manifestation, and that one is the main subject of this article.

Apart from purely 'functional' disorders, the heart is subject to a number of complaints. There are various inflammations, both of its muscular structure, and its containing and lining membranes. Its valvular mechanism may be defective from birth, or be injured through bodily disease. Some of these conditions have been described elsewhere in this book. Comparatively few forms of heart disease cause pain, and many do not seriously threaten life—indeed, a perfectly sound heart is probably rather a rarity, like perfect eyesight. Even angina pectoris, which certainly cannot be regarded lightly, is by no means necessarily fatal—many people who have it in some degree lead tolerably comfortable lives for years.

Angina pectoris is not strictly a disease of the heart itself but of a blood-vessel which feeds the heart-muscle, the 'coronary artery'. The name means simply 'chest pain', which, of course, is not a disease but a symptom. But although its effect on the heart is, so to speak, secondary, the connexion is so fundamental that for all practical purposes we may call it a disease of the heart. The heart is related to the blood-stream in two different ways. First, it is the pumping apparatus which drives the blood through the body. The heart itself derives no direct nourishment from the main blood-stream which merely passes through it; but since, like other pieces of mechanism, it cannot function without fuel, its muscles must have a blood-supply of their own. This blood is supplied from the general circulation through vessels known as the coronary arteries. If these arteries are diseased, the heart's nutrition suffers; if they cease to maintain a normal supply of blood, heart failure follows.

Such an interruption of the 'pipe-line' occurs in the condition called 'coronary thrombosis' described elsewhere in this book. In thrombosis the artery is blocked by a clot, and as this is a sudden disaster, immediate death frequently results. In angina there is no such blockage, but there is a narrowing of the artery which reduces—or in extreme cases cuts off altogether—the supply of blood to the heart-muscle. The actual cause of this narrowing is not fully understood. Obviously, disease of the coronary arteries themselves, or general disease of the body predisposing to arterial disease, can narrow the 'bore' of these vessels. Hardening of their walls, which makes them inelastic and therefore unyielding to the 'thrust' of the volume of blood passing through them has such an effect, and can be a consequence of certain chronic diseases such as rheumatism. Advancing age, which is generally accompanied by degeneration of the walls of the blood-vessels, is a factor. The consequences of these and other conditions, presumably deriving from different causes, can be covered by the expression 'angina pectoris', but there is not as yet general agreement as to how to classify them. An actual attack of angina may, also, be linked with something which causes a spasmodic contraction of the coronary artery, closing it completely.

An attack gives the victim no warning. He experiences a sudden pain in the chest of great intensity, which rapidly becomes agonizing, perhaps spreading to other regions—down the left arm is common. The chest feels as if tightly gripped, breathing is difficult, and movement impossible. The face may turn very pale, and usually has an expression of great anxiety, for the sufferer often feels a sensation as of impending death. The attack does not last long—seconds or minutes, according to its severity—but while it lasts it is most alarming to the patient and distressing to the beholders. Many sufferers live for years after their first attack; but usually the attacks occur at shorter intervals as the disease progresses, they tend to become more severe and their after-effects last longer, until the time comes when the attack is fatal.

Much can be done to palliate the symptoms. Drugs which cause the blood-vessels to dilate are obviously a rational remedy. Nitro-glycerine (the same substance as the explosive, but the medicinal dose is exceedingly small—perhaps as little as a two-hundredth of a grain) is swallowed, and the vapour of a liquid called amyl nitrite is inhaled, both giving instant relief. Recently, attempts have been made to cure the disease by means of a surgical operation. It is too early to speak with confidence about this procedure, but many wonderful operations on the heart itself have now become practicable which would have been thought incredible only a few years ago.

The anginal patient can do much to help himself. As it is evident that his coronary arteries are not capable of bearing the extra load occasioned by any undue strain, he must avoid exertions likely to impose such strains. An attack may be provoked by apparently trifling causes such as the effort of walking uphill or against a strong wind, exposure to cold, and the like. And in angina, as in other heart diseases, mental effort may have as serious consequences as physical. Anxiety, restlessness, undue excitement, lack of tranquil environment, all are to be avoided—unfortunately this is advice easier to give than to carry out.

APOPLEXY (*STROKE*)

To many families the announcement that a relative—usually an elderly person—has 'had a stroke' is a frightening one. What then is the nature of the disaster? The essential feature is injury to the brain, and the commonest cause of this injury is the breaking of a small blood-vessel with resultant bleeding into the brain-substance, an event known as 'cerebral haemorrhage'. Two consequences follow; first, the blood circulation beyond the point where the break occurred is shut off, and the tissues it should have nourished are starved; second, the oozing of blood from the broken vessel damages the delicate tissues in its neighbourhood. It is easy to understand that such occurrences in so important an organ as the brain are likely to have very serious effects, their extent depending on the severity of the bleeding and its location. Sometimes, though rarely, death follows cerebral haemorrhage almost at once. In some other cases the victim may linger for a time—from hours to days—only to succumb without regaining consciousness. In most of these latter cases the bleeding has continued and perhaps increased in volume, causing great pressure on the brain and ultimate destruction of vital regions.

Apoplexy can occur from causes other than cerebral haemorrhage. In the article which discusses thrombosis there is an allusion to the condition termed 'cerebral thrombosis'; in this, one of the blood-vessels of the brain is blocked by a clot, which shuts off the blood-supply to the part the vessel should serve. This part, deprived of nourishment, ceases to function. Similar consequences follow 'cerebral embolism' in which case the blocking of the vessel has been caused, not by a clot of local origin, but by a fragment which, detached from a clot somewhere else in the body, has floated along in the blood-stream until it has stuck in the narrow bore of a cerebral vessel. There are a few other conditions which can give rise to apoplexy, but these three—haemorrhage, thrombosis, and embolism—are the most likely.

The symptoms of apoplexy vary according to the nature and extent of the mishap in the brain. Some cases of apoplexy (generally those involving haemorrhage) are immediately, or almost immediately, fatal. Usually in cases of haemorrhage the stroke happens quite suddenly—perhaps the victim first feels faint and dizzy, then collapses and becomes unconscious; later symptoms affect breathing and other functions. Where thrombosis or embolism is the cause, the onset is more gradual and generally there is no loss of consciousness. But in most cases where the victim survives, a chief symptom is paralysis. This may be total or partial, slight or extreme. Usually, it is confined to one side of the body—hence it is called 'hemiplegia'—and the side affected is that opposite to the side of the brain where the haemorrhage, thrombosis, or embolism occurred. In very mild cases there may be little more than a paralysis of one side of the face, in bad cases the whole of one side of the body is involved; paralysis extends to the arms, legs, hands, and feet, and the power of speech may be lost or greatly impaired.

Liability to apoplexy is increased by extra fragility of the cerebral blood-vessels, a condition more usual with elderly people, for with advancing age the walls of the blood-vessels tend to lose their elasticity and harden, somewhat like 'perished' rubber tubing. Then, if the pressure of the blood within them increases, their walls, unable to expand sufficiently to meet the extra strain, yield at the weakest place. The smaller the vessels, the more likely they are to break—and there are many exceedingly small vessels in the brain. Again, if a person already suffers from abnormally high blood-pressure (a condition called hypertension and described in another article) the risk of apoplexy is increased. This obtains, too, in certain diseases which cause premature hardening of the arteries. Cerebral thrombosis and cerebral embolism do not necessarily presume hardened arteries; they develop where some condition predisposing to clot-formation exists.

Not very much can be done to treat apoplexy. To prevent its occurrence in persons who are of what our forefathers called a plethoric constitution we can take certain measures —some of these are described in the article on hypertension. When a stroke occurs, the victim must be put to bed and very carefully nursed. In the old days he would have been 'bled', and even today some experienced doctors hold that 'venesection' has its uses, within limits. But everything depends on how much damage has been done to the brain, and often this cannot be assessed until some time after the stroke. The initial paralysis may grow worse, or may pass off, or lessen considerably while leaving some degree of permanent loss of function—for example, in some cases speech is never fully restored, in others there is permanent reduction of mental capacity. Moreover, unless the conditions which brought about the stroke can somehow be improved, there is always the possibility that another may follow, sooner or later. It is not true, as is popularly believed, that a second or third attack is inevitably fatal (as we have seen, a single stroke can be); but it is certainly true that each attack reduces the victim's 'expectation of life'.

PEPTIC ULCER

AN ulcer is popularly thought to be a kind of open sore; but there is rather more to it than that. The process of ulceration is a process of local death of the tissues—'necrosis' is the medical term—which progresses layer by layer, gradually extending and eating away the tissues—somewhat after the fashion of digging a pit. There are many varieties of ulcers, and they arise from many different causes. Most of them have their openings somewhere on the surface of the body, and these appear hollowed-out like miniature bomb-craters. If untreated, they go deeper and deeper, increasing in area and doing much local destruction.

But ulcers are not confined to the surface of the body; the process of ulceration can arise in internal organs too, in particular in the digestive organs. Two regions are specially liable to become ulcerated, the stomach and the duodenum (a short tube, the first stretch of the small intestine leading out of the stomach). Ulcers in either of these regions are known as 'peptic ulcers', though it is still common to distinguish them as gastric and duodenal ulcers respectively.

There are special characteristics of peptic ulcers which we shall discuss later. For the moment we need note only that this form of internal ulceration follows the same course as the external kind, but opening on a surface of 'mucous membrane' instead of skin. The mucous membrane is a very smooth tissue which lines the whole of the digestive tract, from the mouth where food is taken in, all the way to the

external orifice of the bowel whence waste residue is expelled. The stomach and duodenum of course share in this
general lining, which protects them from the action of the
'gastric juice', and so saves them from being themselves
'digested', as is meat which enters a healthy stomach.
Besides acting as a protective lining, the mucous membrane
has several very important functions, among them being the
production of the fluid—'mucus'—from which it takes its
name. This mucus, which has the feel—though not the
appearance—of soapy water, ensures that objects slither
along the surfaces it lubricates, thus protecting the membrane itself from injury by, for example, friction.

Not so very many years ago people thought they knew all
about the stomach and the intestines, and understood the
digestive process. Nowadays we are less sure of our knowledge. We have learned, for instance, that the stomach is
very far from being the simple organ, the passive receptacle
for food undergoing chemical action, that it was once
thought to be. We now realize that it works in a very complicated fashion, involving not only the performance of
chemical and mechanical operations but also a close association with the mind—emotions influence its working very
considerably and even cause it in a manner of speaking to
blush or turn pale! Some fortunate accidents (though probably the subjects did not regard them in that light) have
exposed the interior of human stomachs to direct observation from the outside. This has made it possible to collect
evidence about the differing effects on the stomach brought
about both by the introduction of different substances, and
even by the influence of various states of mind. Through
such series of experiments, correlated with a great deal of
careful study of a less spectacular kind, much valuable information has been accumulated.

Although doctors now fairly clearly understand the

mechanism of ulcer-formation, its ultimate cause, about which numerous theories exist, cannot be regarded as established. Undoubtedly a factor is the acid gastric secretion; it is reasonable to assume that, if conditions arise which allow this secretion to attack the lining of the organs, it will eat away their tissues. Internal ulcers will ensue in much the same way as ordinary ulcers grow in the flesh. Mucous membranes which become swollen and congested are prone to be injured readily by local irritation; if with a slight local abrasion, for example, there is associated a loss of the protective film of mucus, the acid secretion gets to work on the tissues beneath. The process may be likened to an artist's 'etching' on metal, where the surface is coated with a film of wax through which lines are scratched to allow acid to 'bite' into the metal thus exposed.

The effects of peptic ulcers range from the distress of more or less chronic ill health to the peril of most dangerous emergencies. As the ulcer eats its way into the wall of the organ, it is likely to injure a number of small blood-vessels; this may result only in slight internal bleeding (though anaemia can arise from the continual loss of blood); but if the erosion is on a considerable scale, rapid and very serious internal haemorrhage will follow. Another risk is that in time the ulcer may eat (perforate) right through the wall, so that the pit becomes bottomless, in short there is a hole through which the contents of the stomach or duodenum leak out into the abdominal cavity to cause 'peritonitis'.

Happily, ulcers are not often nowadays neglected long enough for these acute conditions to develop, but the chronic kind still cause much suffering. They are so painful that victims of gastric ulcer often dread the consequences of taking food (in duodenal ulcer the pain may be relieved by eating, but soon recurs), with the result that they lose weight and become weak and unfit for either work or play. Ulcers may heal of their own accord, but, if they do, they leave scars in the tissues which may become the seat of later trouble. It is an interesting fact that, whereas formerly gastric ulcers were common and duodenal ulcers comparatively rare, nowadays the reverse is the case; duodenal ulcer is on the increase, and the majority of its victims are men (about four times as many men as women are affected). There is no doubt at all that mental strain has a great deal to do with this. Anxieties of the kind which modern life provokes are very apt, in people of a 'worrying' disposition, to produce just those changes in the mucous membranes which prepare the way for the onset of an ulcer.

Unfortunately, recommendations not to worry are usually counsels of perfection. Ulcers do afflict people, and doctors have to do something about it. Formerly there was not a great deal that could be done, except administer palliatives. In really bad cases surgeons cut out the ulcerated parts— a drastic remedy which did not necessarily effect a permanent cure, for it did not prevent another ulcer starting up in a fresh place. Surgical procedures, however, were often essential to deal with such complications as severe haemorrhage or perforation—indeed, the need for the surgeon's aid has by no means disappeared today. Nevertheless, methods have been discovered whereby many peptic ulcers can be cured without operation; they consist of a combination of a very carefully planned diet with the administration of certain drugs which directly influence gastric secretion and the movements of the stomach. If these methods are pursued for a certain length of time, the ulcer heals. Incidentally, it is of interest to note that in some cases it is possible to effect healing without any drugs at all; though much depends on the cause of the ulcer (so far as that can be ascertained) and the temperament of the patient.

Here it is necessary to utter a word of warning. No

attempt should be made at self-medication for ulcer, or indeed for any condition involving the digestive system. There is no panacea: individual diagnosis is vital to treatment, and only a properly qualified doctor is competent to make the examinations which are the essential preliminary.

APPENDICITIS

THE digestive tract consists of the stomach and the intestines, or bowels. The latter, although a continuous tube, are classified anatomically into 'small' and 'large' segments. The first part of the small intestine, that which immediately adjoins the stomach, is known as the 'duodenum'; it continues as the 'jejunum', and that in turn as the 'ileum'. The ileum opens into a sort of cave, pouch, or lobby called the 'caecum', from which leads the large intestine—the 'colon', leading to the 'rectum'. Attached to the caecum, opening into it at one end and closed at the other, is a short, narrow tube a few inches in length; this is the 'vermiform appendix', and when it is inflamed the condition is termed appendicitis.

The appendix is a 'vestigial' organ, that is to say, it serves no useful purpose now, though doubtless it did for man's remote ancestors with their different feeding habits. Nowadays its only importance is as a common site of disease. Incidentally, it is wrong to say, as is sometimes said, that appendicitis is a modern disease unheard of until a royal illness of fifty years ago. The name had not, indeed, up to then been generally adopted, but the condition was well known under a variety of masquerades such as 'perityphlitis': in fact, much of the 'inflammation of the bowels' spoken of by doctors for centuries past must really have been appendicitis.

As the appendix is a cul-de-sac, it has a natural tendency

to collect odd scraps of matter from adjacent parts of the intestines. Once in, they cannot easily get out. Very small fruit-seeds, toothbrush-bristles, and other foreign objects tend to collect there, and some of the normal contents of the bowel (which should pass along to the large intestine to be expelled from the body) flow into the appendix, hardening there into lumps called 'faecal concretions'. Such contents may not of themselves be actively harmful, but they nearly always carry with them micro-organisms which infect the lining of the walls of the appendix. This lining may be infected in another way. If any organisms of disease happen to be in the blood-stream, they will easily infect an appendix irritated by debris lodged in it with consequent weakening of the resistance of its tissues.

Appendicitis, therefore, is the inflammatory reaction provoked by a local infection. If it is confined to the innermost lining, the mucous membrane, the result is a mild chronic inflammation, the so-called 'grumbling appendix', of which the symptoms are vague pains in the abdomen, with some indigestion and perhaps a feeling of nausea. These symptoms may last a long time, or may subside. A great many people in the past, before abdominal surgery was sufficiently advanced, probably suffered from chronic appendicitis and recovered without treatment. But the chronic form can, and frequently does, 'light up' suddenly and develop into the acute form, and that is not likely to have a happy ending of its own accord.

Acute appendicitis is a serious condition usually calling for urgent operation. Its first symptom, severe pain in the abdomen, may not be felt in the region of the appendix, but more toward the centre, even round the navel. In fact, the appendix is not always in the same place in different individuals, and so the old advice for locating it—'with the right hand in the trouser pocket, the thumb covers the appendix'—is not wholly reliable. Later on, however, the pain is definitely felt on the right side, rather low down. There will probably be some vomiting, and most likely complete constipation, though in certain cases the opposite condition—diarrhoea—may arise. There will be some fever, and if the abdomen is felt expertly round the region of the appendix, it will be found 'rigid' but tender to the touch.

Even an acute attack of appendicitis may pass off, but the risks of awaiting the event (which the odds are against) are too great to justify. For if the process of inflammation spreads, it involves the whole of the appendix and perhaps the neighbouring parts. An abscess may form, suppurate, and burst into the abdominal cavity. This is one cause of the condition known as 'perforation' of the appendix. The appendix is, as we have said, normally a closed tube except where it joins the caecum; but, if it perforates, it is to all intents and purposes just a hole in the bowel, through which the contents of the latter leak out continuously into the abdominal cavity. As the escaping matter is infective, the very dangerous condition of 'peritonitis'—general inflammation of the lining of the abdomen—follows, and calls for emergency surgery if the patient's life is to be saved.

The only treatment of acute appendicitis, whether it has reached these graver stages or not, is surgical excision of the appendix and the closure of the gap in the caecum left by its removal. Modern surgery has made this a very simple procedure, and most of the risks which formerly existed have been removed by the use of the sulphonamides and antibiotics, which singly or in combination control infection. If perforation has developed, however, the patient may be very severely 'shocked' and in a bad state to undergo operation. The rule therefore is to operate at once after acute appendicitis has been diagnosed.

Appendicitis occurs at all ages, but most frequently before

middle life, and it is quite common in children and young people. Removal of the appendix is, of course, a complete cure, and persons without an appendix are absolutely unaffected in all respects. These facts are so well established that there have been cases of people having their appendixes removed without any urgent necessity, merely because they intended to travel in remote or primitive countries where surgical emergencies could not so easily be dealt with. But perhaps that is carrying foresight a little too far!

ARTHRITIS

THIS word which, strictly, ought to denote conditions involving inflammation of joints, has come to be used rather loosely and may now refer to a number of conditions which our forefathers called 'rheumatism', or more commonly 'the screws'. There are a whole lot of these conditions, their manifestations ranging from an occasional twinge to a crippling malady which renders the victim bedridden and completely helpless. This group of diseases is so widespread —in Britain, it has been estimated, about half the population over the age of 40 suffer from them in varying degree—that an international organization has been formed to combat them.

Perhaps we had better begin by classifying these different types of arthritis, though, even among doctors, there is considerable dispute on this question, since patients often display a complication of various types. First, there is arthritis properly so called, the affection of the joints. (Statements in the article on Sprains, Strains, and Dislocations about the construction and normal working of joints should be referred to now.) Arthritis, properly so called, can arise from anything which causes local inflammation—it can cer-

tainly be caused by various general diseases such as tuberculosis and gonorrhoea. But when we speak of arthritis as
a specific disease, we generally mean a chronic condition of
either 'rheumatoid arthritis' or 'osteo-arthritis'.

Rheumatoid arthritis which manifests itself only in the
joints, is really a 'systemic' disease, that is to say, the whole
body is affected though the symptoms are chiefly local. The
patient is really suffering from the disease before he or she
(women are the more usual sufferers) knows about it.
Joints, as we read later in this book, are surrounded by
various 'soft tissues', and it is these tissues which first become
inflamed. The inflammation spreads inwards towards the
moving parts of the joint, till the smooth working together
of the bones is destroyed, and the joint gradually 'seizes up',
as an engineer would say. When the joint cannot be moved,
the muscles which serve it gradually waste away, and swellings of increasing size appear around the joints. Of course
pain is associated with these local changes, and the patient's
general health is much affected. The disease may in course
of time extend to all the joints in the body, even to those of
the spine.

Osteo-arthritis is a different condition which, unlike
rheumatoid arthritis, is commoner in males than in females.
It really is a local disease. It affects, not the soft tissues surrounding the joint, but the surfaces of the ends of the bones
(which, in the 'rheumatoid' variety, are not affected until a
later stage). In osteo-arthritis the cartilage which normally
covers the ends of the bones wears away at the places where
the joint is subjected to most pressure, for just the same reason that a sock gets a hole in the heel. Once the cartilage has
thus started to wear, it is gradually rubbed away until the
bare bones are left just grating together. Naturally, this
makes the joint work stiffly. But there is another reason for
stiffness, too, in that a local reaction causes 'overgrowths'

of bone which result in a locking-up of the joint similar in kind though not in cause to that in the late stages of rheumatoid arthritis. Osteo-arthritis likewise causes pain and muscle-wasting, but, unlike the rheumatoid variety, it usually confines itself to one or two joints, though commonly important ones such as the hips or knees.

But there are many kinds of rheumatic pains which are not localized to the joints and, indeed, may not affect them at all. Strictly this group should not be included under the heading 'arthritis'. Many people complain of what they call 'muscular rheumatism'. There is a kind of inflammation of the muscles, called 'myositis'; but few of the people who feel tenderness or pain in their muscles are suffering from this condition. What they probably have is 'fibrositis', certainly a trying malady, as will be agreed when I instance 'lumbago' as one of its forms, but not really an inflammation of the muscles themselves: when muscular pain is felt it is generally because the fibrous tissue of the muscle-sheath is affected. Fibrositis can affect fibrous tissue anywhere and is known by a variety of names. But naturally it often involves muscles both because most parts of the body have muscles lying somewhere around and because muscles include some fibrous tissue. We need to have clearly in our minds the broad distinction between 'articular' and 'non-articular' rheumatism, remembering that the latter always affects soft tissues, often but not necessarily those anywhere near joints. Next we need to remember the fact that of the two forms of 'articular rheumatism' only one, rheumatoid arthritis, is entitled to be properly so called. The other, osteo-arthritis, is not a 'rheumatic' affection at all, but, as we have seen, a bone affection.

We must give a moment to consider the acute form of rheumatism, or 'rheumatic fever'. As the name implies, this is a disease in which all the symptoms common to rheumatic

affections develop suddenly, rapidly, and severely; after the
disease has run a course of days or weeks, the symptoms subside. While they last, the patient (usually a child or young
adult) experiences all the troubles of the chronic cases
described above, and a few extra ones thrown in. There are
the painful joints—one after another becoming involved—the
swellings, the fibrositis, and in addition there are the special
symptoms of a fever. With modern treatment all these pass
off much more quickly than in former times, but there is
still one serious effect of rheumatic fever which cannot
easily be dealt with—the acute inflammation usually extends to the heart, which may be left permanently damaged.

We have now reached the stage when, as we generally do
in these short accounts of diseases, we can discuss fundamental causes. But we cannot find a complete answer in this
case. There is general agreement that acute rheumatism
(rheumatic fever) is due to infection by some micro-
organism since so much about it is typical of the many
febrile diseases originating thus. As yet, we have not identified the actual organism, nor do we even know if it is an
ordinary germ or a virus. It is possibly an organism of a
commonplace kind which achieves special virulence in certain individuals under unusual conditions.

There can be no doubt that the immediate cause of osteo-
arthritis is the 'mechanical' factor of weight, pressure, and
friction at the end of the bones which form a joint. It is not
so clear why these circumstances, which obviously are liable
to arise in anybody, provoke osteo-arthritis in comparatively
few people. Advancing age is a contributory factor, as are
injuries of various kinds, and possibly, though osteo-
arthritis is essentially a local disease, some general bodily
disorders. On the other hand, the cause of rheumatoid
arthritis is controversial. Until recently two main theories
held the field—one, that the cause was a micro-organism of

some kind (this received support from the accepted fact that such a cause exists in acute rheumatism), the other, that the cause was 'focal sepsis'. Certain parts of the body can harbour permanently various micro-organisms which, while not usually associated with particular diseases, can indirectly cause general disease. The sites where they harbour are known as 'infective foci', and these are, chiefly, the teeth, the appendix, the gall-bladder, the tonsils, and the 'sinuses' (hollow spaces) of the skull—although there are many other possible sites. The infection thus caused is the focal sepsis. But recently an entirely new theory of the origin of rheumatoid arthritis has been put forward, that it may be due to an 'endocrine' disorder, that is to say, to a disturbance of the system of glands which produce internal secretions. We shall return to this point later. As regards fibrositis in its various forms, the main cause is likely to be some kind of focal sepsis, but another cause may be the prolonged strain of an unnatural posture either in work or play, perhaps aggravated by exposure to cold or damp.

What can we do to relieve sufferers? For acute rheumatism (or rheumatic fever) the treatment is more or less that of most fevers—rest in bed under the care of a doctor. The most valuable drugs, which are also useful in some chronic forms of rheumatism, are compounds of 'salicylic acid' (aspirin is one of them). For osteo-arthritis we can do a great deal of good by physical methods—local heat, massage, certain exercises. In bad cases special 'caliper' splints may be needed to enable the patient to walk; in very bad cases surgical operations on the bones of the affected joints may be necessary. An attack of fibrositis yields to a combination of internal and external remedies, the latter including various plasters, poultices, and liniments, special baths, 'infra-red rays', and, finally, exercises.

A specific advance in treatment seems likely now for

rheumatoid arthritis. It has for long been known that women suffering from this disease often experience relief from their symptoms if they become pregnant, and that similar relief is experienced by patients who have an attack of jaundice. Now it happens that in both pregnancy and jaundice a change takes place in the 'internal secretions' of the body, particularly in certain secretions (hormones) of the 'suprarenal glands' (two small organs situated close to the kidneys) and the 'pituitary gland' (a small organ at the base of the brain). The deduction was accordingly made that in rheumatoid arthritis there is some deficiency or altered balance of hormones, and, starting from this hypothesis, it has been discovered that the hormone-balance can be corrected by dosing the patients with compounds called 'ACTH' and 'cortisone', compounds which substitute for the secretions the glands should produce for themselves. Very remarkable results are claimed for these new treatments, but the compounds are as yet so scarce that insufficient experience has been acquired in their use. So far as we can tell, patients who cease to take them relapse, just as diabetics do if deprived of insulin.

We must not conclude our brief survey without mentioning two earlier treatments for rheumatoid arthritis, both of which have their advocates. One is 'vaccine therapy', which is based on the belief that a micro organism is responsible. The other is the use of gold: salts of the metal are dissolved, and the solutions injected into the muscles. Both these treatments have been in use for many years, and are likely to continue in favour until the new treatment described in the preceding paragraph becomes established and available.

DIABETES

FROM very early times a disease was known of which the two most obvious symptoms were habitual thirst and the discharge of unusually large quantities of urine—hence the significance of the name given it by the Greeks. There are in fact two diseases in which these symptoms predominate, and both are called diabetes although their origins are quite different, but whereas one form, diabetes *insipidus*, is usually unaccompanied by any other sign of ill health, the other, diabetes *mellitus*, is a disease with many serious manifestations. Colloquially, 'diabetes' refers to the latter, diabetes *mellitus*, of which we now treat.

Next to excessive flow of urine, its most important characteristic is, as indicated by 'mellitus', the presence in the urine of sugar. There are many kinds of sugar, all members of a particular group of chemical compounds. The kind of sugar present in diabetic urine is glucose. How does it get there, and why does it matter?

It is quite literally true to say that all through our lives we are 'burning up' certain material in our tissues, and this process of combustion provides our bodily heat and our muscular vigour. The oxygen in the air we breathe, the food and water we eat and drink, furnish, among other things, the fuel substance which enables the body to carry on all its activities. The efficiency of the 'fuel' is measured in calories, which are units of heat. Several components of our diet are essential for the preservation of life and health. The chief of these are proteins to build up and repair our tissues, fats to form a reserve stock of energy-providers (as well as fulfilling other physiological functions), and carbohydrates to burn as regular fuel. We also need certain minerals, and of course vitamins. For our present purpose we can concentrate on the carbohydrates. Broadly speaking, carbohydrates are starch-like substances—found chiefly in bread, potatoes, cereals, certain vegetables, and milk—and sugars of all kinds. Now starch as starch is of no use to anybody except a laundress; it has to undergo a process of conversion in our digestive system before it can be used as fuel. Essentially, the process converts all kinds of carbohydrate into sugar, in which form it can be readily burnt up.

Ideally, of course, our intake of carbohydrates, converted into sugar, should balance our output of energy and maintain a small reserve. How is this regulated? Carbohydrate metabolism, as it is technically termed, depends upon the interaction of certain glands of the body, the one principally concerned being the 'pancreas'. This organ, about seven inches long and shaped something like a horizontal letter J, is situated behind the stomach. Butchers and cooks call it the sweetbread. It includes certain very important parts called the 'islets of Langerhans' after the scientist who first observed them. These 'islets' produce a secretion called insulin, whose function is to render usable as fuel the sugar into which our carbohydrate has been converted. Thus the story should run: the digestive organs convert carbohydrates into sugar; insulin makes this sugar available for combustion; the sugar is burned up into energy to supply our bodily needs.

But in some people the pancreas fails, suddenly or gradually, to produce insulin. When this happens, although all the other stages of carbohydrate metabolism have been completed, the final and vital stage has not. The carbohydrate has been turned into sugar, and the sugar is circulating in the blood just as it ought to be, but the insulin is not there to free it for use by the tissues. So the sugar stays in the blood, doing no useful service, until, in the course of filtration through the kidneys, it passes into the urine and is lost altogether. Now the body, deprived of its fuel, weakens and wastes. The patient acquires persistent thirst and that frequency of urination that gives diabetes its name. He (or she, though the disease is much commoner in men) loses weight, becomes exhausted quickly, and suffers in many other ways. If untreated, the sufferer would die—probably in a comatose state.

Until about thirty years ago, the only treatment known was a very rigorous restriction of diet. As diabetes was obviously a disorder of carbohydrate metabolism, the patient was forbidden practically all food containing starch or sugar. This, of course, by depriving him of a main source of energy, greatly restricted his activities. If a child developed diabetes, the outlook was very grave; for, although he might just manage to get along on his meagre diet, he had no surplus to provide for his rapid growth. Consequently, the diabetic child rarely lived to reach manhood. Happily all that is now changed by the discovery that insulin obtained from other sources could be supplied to patients who were unable to manufacture it for themselves. If all that was previously lacking was insulin, and that lack was compensated, the diabetic became as good as the next man. But the administration of insulin does not cure diabetes; it does not help the body to make any for itself. We still do not know what has gone wrong with the pancreas to cause its insulin production to cease, and, until we find this out, we cannot say we have cured diabetes. Moreover, as insulin cannot be swallowed (if it is, the digestive juices destroy it), the diabetic must suffer it to be injected beneath the skin, usually at least once every day throughout life. Diet too, although no longer the essential feature of treatment, is still very important. But insulin, together with dieting, enables the diabetic to live a fairly normal life, and has enormously reduced the death-rate, especially of children. Its introduction was one of the greatest advances in medicine.

THYROID DEFICIENCY AND EXCESS

FROM time to time throughout these articles I have mentioned the 'endocrine system' and the 'hormones' which it produces. This exceedingly important subject has brought into existence a whole new branch of medicine, 'endocrinology'. I propose now to discuss a typical endocrine organ, but before doing so it is necessary to speak of the system in general. Briefly, it consists of certain glands which, situated at various places in the body, secrete substances profoundly affecting our physiological functions. The body has many glands which are not of endocrine nature; these also produce secretions which they pour into the organ they serve through 'ducts'. The endocrine glands, on the other hand, have no ducts, and so are sometimes called the 'ductless' glands. Their secretions pass directly into the circulating blood by way of the small vessels which traverse the glands; they are sometimes described as 'internal secretions', but are now more usually called 'hormones'.

The hormones are chemical substances of great complexity, which act almost like artificial medicinal substances taken into the body. That is to say, a hormone, after it has got out of its parent gland into the blood-stream, travels to the part of the body where it is to exert its special influence, and does just that job and no more. The hormones perform very varied tasks; they regulate growth both before and after birth, they control metabolism (the conversion into energy of food, &c., taken into the body), they order sexual development and sex activity, blood-pressure, the excretion of urine, and many other essential functions. Certain of the endocrine organs are truly vital in that life cannot exist in their absence. Others, although not vital in this sense, are so essential that, if the body is without them, it is affected by serious disease. An example of the effects of hormone deficiency is the production of diabetes through lack of the hormone insulin (see p. 92).

Among the endocrine organs one of the most important, the 'thyroid gland', is of particular interest because it was the first of these organs whose function we perceived. From that point the clinical applications of endocrinology began, and through the systematic study of other glands we are now able to understand and treat many diseases which formerly baffled us. The thyroid gland is situated in the front of the neck, below what is commonly called the 'Adam's apple', partly surrounding the windpipe or 'trachea'. In adults its average length is about two inches, its width slightly more than its length, its thickness about one inch. Usually, though not always, it is divided into two 'lobes' which are connected by a bridge of tissue. Its function is to manufacture a hormone called 'thyroxin', which it conveys directly into the blood-stream.

Leaving the gland itself for a moment, we will consider the following facts. For very many years certain severe diseases had been observed whose causation was unknown. One of these was called 'cretinism' because its victims in some European countries where it was prevalent were termed *cretins*, a French word implying imbecility. These unfortunates were dwarfs of hideous visage, often deaf mutes, always more or less mentally defective; they were born so, and they remained in that state throughout their lives. Another baffling disease was 'myxoedema', which usually affected middle-aged persons. The victims gradually became sluggish and inert, their weight increased, their speech became slow, their memories poor; their hair fell out, their skins coarsened, their features became gross, their expression dull. Then there was the very common condition called 'goitre' in which big uncomfortable swellings developed in the neck—and which seemed particularly rife in certain districts (thus in England 'Derbyshire neck' was a popular synonym). A very severe form was 'exophthalmic goitre' or 'Graves's Disease', now more accurately termed 'primary thyrotoxicosis', characterized by serious loss of weight, a nervous tremor, rapid action of the heart, emotional upsets, and the peculiar appearance of the eyes 'starting from their sockets', which gave the disease one of its names. In some very bad cases the patient died of heart failure; in others the nervous and emotional disturbances developed into acute insanity. Thyrotoxicosis is much more frequent in women than in men, the ratio having been put at six to one.

Strange as it may seem, it is now established that all these diseases, with their very different symptoms and effects, are due to thyroid gland disorders which result in either a deficiency or an excess of production of thyroxin. This hormone, one of the most important products of the endocrine system, has special influence on growth and development. In cretinism the thyroid gland is either absent from birth, or non-functioning, and so there is no thyroxin in the body. In myxoedema the thyroid, previously normal, has degenerated, with the result that thyroxin is produced in insufficient quantity to maintain the proper balance of bodily functions. Ordinary goitre is an enlargement of the gland not usually accompanied with any severe general disturbances of the system. The swelling may, however, by pressing on vital structures in the neck such as the veins, the windpipe, or the gullet, cause discomfort or worse. Although the thyroid is enlarged in goitre, this does not mean that it is more active —on the contrary; for it is the part of the gland which does not produce thyroxin which has over-developed. The enlargement is because insufficient iodine, the essential component of thyroxin, has been taken into the body, and this explains why goitre is especially common in certain districts where iodine is lacking in the soil and water. Thyrotoxicosis differs from all the other conditions mentioned in that it is due to over-activity of the thyroid, producing an excessive outpouring of thyroxin into the blood. The hormone, normally beneficent and, indeed, necessary to life and health, has become through excess a poison.

Once the fundamental relationship between the thyroid gland and these several disorders was understood, effective methods of treatment were speedily devised. It was found that the thyroid glands of animals such as sheep were so similar to ours that various preparations from their glands could be readily assimilated by patients with results equalling those of their own glands, had they been functioning. In cretinism the results were so dramatic as to appear miraculous—the stunted, dwarfish, mute, imbecile child began to develop normally, its stature grew, it learned to speak, its mental state improved; in short, it became capable of ordinary existence. For as long as it continued to receive thyroid treatment, this continued; if treatment was stopped, the condition relapsed, because the child was still incapable of producing thyroxin for itself. Myxoedema was similarly treated with equally beneficial results—here too, generally speaking, the patient has to continue the treatment indefinitely. With goitre, treatment usually takes the form of surgical removal of part of the swollen gland, if the symptoms of pressure are so distressing as to justify operation. But it is in the prevention of goitre that the most notable advance has been made: in districts where iodine is naturally lacking, it is administered to the population usually in the form of iodized table salt, and this small daily dose from early life onward is sufficient to prevent ordinary goitres from developing.

Thyrotoxicosis, as already indicated, comes into a different category, although, as in goitre, there is enlargement of the thyroid gland. The cause of primary thyrotoxicosis is not known, but, as its essential feature is an excessive production of thyroxin, what is clearly needed is something to reduce the secretion. Formerly the most effective means of accomplishing this was to remove part or even the whole of the thyroid gland surgically (if the whole was removed the patient had to take thyroid extract thereafter to prevent myxoedema—a going from one extreme to the other). Other methods were also used to reduce the size of the gland, and hence of its thyroxin output. X-rays and radium have been used—indeed, all these treatments are still used in special cases, and a number of medicinal treatments have been in vogue in the past, with varying success. One has recently been discovered which is both more potent and more 'rational' than any which have gone before. It is the administration of a substance called 'thiouracil', which gains its end by stopping the production of thyroxin (what it actually does is prevent the building-up or synthesis of the thyroxin molecule from iodine by the thyroid gland). An even more remarkable treatment is now being used. One of the 'radioactive isotopes' (by-products of nuclear fission, which are ordinary elements rendered temporarily capable of emitting radiations), is 'radioactive iodine'. This is taken by the mouth, and makes its way to the thyroid gland (its progress can be traced), where it stays. There its radiations, bombarding the tissues of the gland, cause them to shrink, thus checking the over-secretion of thyroxin and curing the thyrotoxicosis.

MENTAL DISEASE

'THE accused was labouring under such a defect of reason from disease of the mind as not to know the nature and quality of the act he was doing; or if he did know it, he did not know he was doing what was wrong.' This extract from the celebrated *McNaghten Rules* indicates the grounds on which, in law, a plea of insanity as a defence to an accusation of wrongdoing must be founded. What, then, is the nature of this 'disease of the mind'?

The brain is the seat of the mind. It is a physical structure —of infinite complexity indeed, yet capable of being separated into parts and minutely examined, like any other organ of the body. By studying the structure of other organs we have gained much knowledge of their method of functioning; but our understanding of how the brain works is still very limited. The brain is the control-tower of the body, which regulates all the movements of our limbs, &c., and we know precisely which parts of it control our bodily activities. More, we know just whereabouts in the brain reside the receiving-stations of our senses. We can identify the areas respectively concerned with almost every physiological function. But when we have done all this, there remains a large region—located chiefly in the 'frontal lobes' —which we understand very little about. We can only surmise that here if anywhere is the seat of those qualities of our being which appear to have nothing to do with the body— memory, imagination, judgement, beliefs, emotions—all the intangibles which go to make up the personality. Are these, too, functions of matter? To this question, one of the most profoundly important in life, many men have given different answers. Here we can say only that, so far as our human experience goes, 'mind' is found only in association with 'brain', and the brain is a physical structure.

We have said that the 'motor' and 'sensory' areas of the brain can be easily located. It may be supposed that any injury to these areas must affect the bodily functions which they control. This is so—indeed, by observing the effects of injuries we have gained knowledge of the relation of these areas to their respective functions. But how do the areas themselves normally co-operate, as it were, in enabling us to live our lives? We know that some of their functioning is automatic, controlled by a system of 'reflexes' which is not much more difficult to understand than is the working of an automatic telephone exchange. But with most of the complicated operations of our daily lives, there is much more to it than automatic function. For example, we are driving a car along a road when we see a threatened danger. We steer away from it, accelerate or slow down, or stop the car, as the case may be—all actions which appear to us practically automatic and instantaneous. But what actually has happened? An optical image has been projected by the lens of the eye upon the retina (see p. 115). It is transmuted into nerve-impulses which reach the brain via the optic nerve. The brain interprets these impulses as impressions of external things. Now comes a gap in the narration which we will pass over for the moment to go straight on to the next stage. In this stage, the motor areas of the brain responsible for the control of muscles send their orders to the hands and feet to move the steering-wheel, to raise or depress the accelerator pedal, perhaps to take out the clutch, put on the brakes, and move the gear level into neutral.

A good driver does all these things, he believes, automatically. He would say that he doesn't need to think, he acts as if he were part of the machine. With all respect to him, he is mistaken—the fact is that his experience has taught him to think fast and to act very rapidly so that his 'reaction time' is very short, but he has had to go through all the motions just the same. And the most important stage in the train of work is the 'gap' which, in the preceding paragraph, we agreed to pass over. The brain received its message from the eye, and subsequently sent its orders to the muscles. But what determined the nature of the orders? Obviously, the driver, after receiving the danger-signal, made a judgement—a judgement to which his memory of similar experiences, his imagination, his temperament— which may be cautious or reckless, decisive or hesitant, even humane or callous, &c.—all contributed. In short, he made up his mind and, having made it up, acted. Although all this happens extremely quickly, no step in the long train of mental processes can be skipped.

The practical effect of the working of the mind, as in this example, applies to every action of our lives. From playing cricket to committing murder it is the same story: mind controls brain, brain controls body, body acts on environ- ment. (The precise relationship of mind and brain is open to argument, but that does not affect our present purpose.) The normal person's resultant acts are rational, they 'make sense'; but unhappily all persons are not normal. In them something has gone amiss with that higher faculty of the brain which links the inner man to the outer world. All the 'mechanical' parts may continue to function, but the cap- tain, so to speak, has abandoned the bridge. He may never have been there—perhaps before birth some essential part of the brain failed to develop, so that the child was born an idiot, incapable of thought. Less severe forms of congenital defect cause mental deficiency in varying degree. Besides congenital defect, many other things may cause a state of mental disease, temporary or permanent. Bodily disease may extend to the brain: tumours may invade it, drugs in- jure it, or wounds destroy its tissues. But in very many cases of what is commonly termed 'insanity' there is no detectable alteration in the structure of the brain, nothing physical to account for the fact that the individual does not behave like a reasonable person. Doubtless the explanation is to be found, did we know how to seek for it, in that mysterious frontal region to which no definite function can be assigned.

Insanity takes many forms, from the mildness of 'melancholia' to the violence of 'mania'; from the delusions of 'paranoia' to the 'split mind' of 'schizophrenia'. Intermediate forms are numerous, and there are many others which do not fall into any of these categories. This is not the place to give harrowing descriptions of these distressing afflictions. But it is perhaps fitting to dispose of certain misconceptions. First, although for their own safety the insane must be segregated, only a small proportion are dangerous to society. Second, by no means all afflicted persons are hopelessly insane—an increasing number of cases are being cured and restored to normal life. Conditions governing the care of the insane today bear no resemblance to those that prevailed even as recently as the latter part of the nineteenth century when Charles Reade published *Hard Cash*; and long before Reade's time the inhumanity of an earlier day, the 'bedlams' with their chains, whips, and starvation, belonged to a forgotten past. The 'mental hospital' now cares for sufferers from 'diseases of the mind' just as an orthopaedic hospital cares for those with injured limbs.

Until recently, even though mental hospitals employed humane and enlightened methods, they did not possess specific means of treating insanity. Since often, as we remarked above, no physical change accounts for the mental disorder, it did not seem likely that any physical treatment could be effectual. Nevertheless, important advances have been made along these lines, although we do not fully understand how or why some of the new treatments work so well— they are, we say, 'empiric'. Perhaps the most interesting is a surgical operation on the brain termed 'leucotomy'. Of course, brain surgery is not new—it has for long been used to remedy definite physical conditions, as, for example, to remove tumours; but leucotomy is not performed for any such reason. We noted earlier that the frontal lobes, the seat of the higher 'psychical' faculties of the brain, are not, so far as we can tell, differentiated into regions, each with a special faculty; these faculties are diffused throughout the whole— a unique phenomenon. But the frontal lobes are connected to other parts of the brain by 'association pathways', and if these paths are interrupted (either accidentally, or deliberately as in the leucotomy operation) the personality of the individual will change. Leucotomy is suitable only for certain cases, and the changes it produces have not always been beneficial; but it has helped many people to live in comparative freedom from the misery of their previous state.

Another recent treatment is the so-called 'shock therapy'. In illness, accident, or surgery, the physical condition called 'shock' is a serious complication (those who worked in civil defence during the last war will remember how important it was to combat shock in the injured), but it has been found that, in certain types of insanity, the patient can be greatly benefited by shock. It is therefore deliberately induced— strangely enough by the injection of 'insulin', the indispensable remedy for diabetes (see p. 92). In general, the object is to put the patient into a comatose state. A succession of such treatments often greatly improves his mental condition.

Shock therapy is sometimes confused with 'convulsive therapy', probably because of inexact appreciation of the medical meaning of the word 'shock'. In convulsive therapy too, the object is eventually to produce the comatose state, but as the name suggests, only after the patient has experienced a fit resembling an epileptic seizure (see p. 108).

This treatment can be carried out by the use of certain drugs, but many doctors prefer to employ electrical methods.

It is interesting to recall a pioneer effort, still successfully employed, to treat 'general paralysis of the insane' (see p. 19) by giving the patient an artificially-induced fever—deliberate infection with malaria, for example. This 'pyrexial therapy' is really another instance of physical treatment of mental disease; but we should remember that 'G.P.I.' can be definitely ascribed to a physical cause—syphilis. There are several other kinds of treatment nowadays for the relief of insanity, but space permits us to mention only one other, 'continuous narcosis'. In this, drugs are used to keep the patient in a deep slumber almost all the time until his mental condition improves.

Enough has been said to show that insanity can now be actively treated, that we need no longer passively resign ourselves to the hope that nature will work a cure in time, or, worse, believe that once persons become mentally unsound they must remain incurably so all their lives. Continuous and vigorous research has revealed much, though very much more remains to be discovered. But the time may well come when the words with which I opened this article will be of little more than historical interest.

MENINGITIS

THE brain and its continuation the spinal cord, which together form the 'central nervous system', lie within the skull and the bony canal of the spine enclosed in three successive layers of membrane called the 'meninges', much as a fragile parcel is wrapped first in tissue paper, then in white paper, and finally in stout brown paper over all. The meninges, especially the two inner membranes, are liable to inflammation from a variety of causes, and this condition is known as 'meningitis'.

Inflammation can reach the meningeal membranes directly, for example through a wound exposing them to contamination with foreign matter from outside the body. They may also become infected through the proximity of septic matter already in the body, for example in an abscess or an 'infective focus' (see p. 90). But the commonest cause of meningitis is infection of the membranes through micro-organisms carried in the blood-stream, and any one of several different organisms can be concerned in this. One of these is the 'meningococcus', but the organisms of other definite diseases may be responsible, for example those of tuber-culosis, syphilis, and pneumonia; when the meningitis arises from external wound-infection or internal suppuration, the germs ordinarily producing these conditions are guilty.

There is a general similarity between all forms of menin-gitis, however caused. We will describe a case of the menin-gococcal kind as typical. The first symptoms likely to be noticed are severe headache, stiffness of the neck, vomiting, and fever, all coming on suddenly; a little later the patient's mind becomes confused, he may be delirious, he finds light painful to the eyes; later still the limbs begin to stiffen, the backbone arches inwards, the head is pushed back. As the inflammation of the meninges increases, an 'exudate', as such internal discharges are called, flows from them; this causes pressure on the brain and affects the 'cranial' nerves, so that the sufferer may become deaf or blind, temporarily or permanently. Inflammation may spread to the brain itself, causing the condition termed 'encephalitis'. The skin may develop a kind of rash caused by small patches of blood beneath—it is this symptom which gave the name 'spotted fever' to one form of the disease.

Tuberculous and syphilitic meningitis do not usually arise

so suddenly, which is understandable as, in these cases, the inflammation of the meninges has ensued from a pre-existing disease. The other forms of meningitis differ according to their nature in the rapidity of their onset and course. All forms are extremely serious, and until recently were frequently fatal—the tuberculous form invariably so. Meningococcal meningitis (cerebro-spinal fever) is infectious, and tends to run in epidemics. The micro-organism responsible may harbour in the throat and nose of persons who themselves show no sign of illness—they are, we say, 'carriers'. If these carriers, by sneezing, coughing, &c., scatter the germs, other people inhaling them may become ill, as described above. Children are more liable to infection than adults, and epidemics are commoner in the winter than in the summer months. These remarks, it will be understood, relate to the meningococcal form of meningitis—the pneumonial, tuberculous, and syphilitic forms obviously can occur at any season and affect persons of all ages, as of course can meningitis caused by wound-infection or focal sepsis.

Until recent years the treatment of meningitis was unsatisfactory and the death-rate was high. Where the responsible micro-organism was identifiable it was possible to prepare a serum for injection, and this had some success. Various surgical operations were devised for the opening-up of infected areas of the body, and fluid was withdrawn from the spine by 'lumbar puncture'. Incidentally, all these measures have a certain place in treatment at the present day, and have not been utterly superseded. But the whole treatment of meningitis has been transformed by chemotherapy and antibiosis. The first great advance was made with the discovery that members of the 'sulphonamide' group of drugs were specific in the meningococcal form of the disease. Then came 'penicillin', which was equally potent in dealing with the pneumococcal form. This antibiotic is also of great value in dealing with meningococcal meningitis when the latter is associated with a 'toxaemia' (a state of general poisoning of the tissues of the body through disease) with which the sulphonamides cannot deal. Perhaps the most remarkable achievement, however, is the cure of tuberculous meningitis by another antibiotic, 'streptomycin', for this form of the disease was considered absolutely fatal until quite recently, since no case of recovery had ever been recorded. Syphilitic meningitis results from the assault of *Treponema pallidum*, the organism causing syphilis (see p. 17), on the central nervous system. It can nevertheless be treated with penicillin, supplemented perhaps by general 'anti-syphilitic' treatment. Other forms of meningitis, those caused by the organisms of wound-infection or sepsis within the body, can be treated by sulphonamides, or penicillin, or other antibiotics, according to the nature of the hostile organisms. Thus has medical science removed yet another 'killer' from the list of human diseases, and that within the lifetime of the youngest readers of this book.

EPILEPSY

THE connexion between the science of 'electronics' and the study of the human body is not at first obvious. It is not easy to believe that the ordinary radio valve has helped us to a greater understanding of our own vital processes; but so it is. Through its power of amplifying minute electrical impulses so as to make them perceptible to our senses, the valve has started us on the road to some remarkable discoveries.

One of the most mysterious of the many problems confronting physiologists is that of nervous activity. Our brains consist of millions of cells of very special form, and these cells are connected to nerve-fibres which, traversing the entire body, control all our movements and convey all kinds of sensations to our minds or brains. Long ago, men guessed that electricity had something to do with this, for the analogy of the conduction of impulses along nerves with that of electric currents along wires was too striking to be overlooked. But it is dangerous to pursue analogies too far; we know now that a nerve impulse, although certainly accompanied by electrical changes, is much more complicated than a simple electrical phenomenon.

Within the brain, too, there is electrical activity, produced by—to use the language of the physics laboratory—'differences of potential' in the cell tissues. Since these changes in the electrical state of the brain are very minute, the radio valve now comes into the picture. By means of a special apparatus attached to the head, the tiny currents set up by the brain's working are passed through a high-power amplifier and are made to write a record in the form of a graph. This graph is called an 'electro-encephalogram', or E.E.G. for short.

Some extraordinary facts have been established from the study of these graphs. Their normal 'curves' are affected in one way by mental concentration, and in another way by relaxation as in sleep. (But if the sleeper dreams, the rhythm is changed again.) And the graphs also show abnormal curves in certain disorders of the nervous system, of which the most important is epilepsy.

'The falling sickness', as our forefathers called epilepsy, is a sad affliction, and a person in an epileptic fit is a very distressing sight. In the severer type he loses consciousness and falls to the ground, possibly injuring himself, since he has had no time to take precautions; he is thrown into convulsions which, when they pass off, leave him unconscious. The best that can be said is that the fit lasts for only a couple

of minutes and leaves the sufferer with no recollection whatever of the event. He never knows when he is going to have
another attack, for although before a fit he might experience a peculiar sensation known as the 'aura', this
comes too late to be of service as a warning. It is obvious that
a person liable to epileptic seizures must avoid all situations
where a temporary unconsciousness might be dangerous—
he must never ride a bicycle, drive a car, climb a ladder,
swim, or the like. There is a less severe form in which the
sufferer does not fall or suffer convulsions, and in which the
unconsciousness is so transitory that it is almost unnoticed;
but this form has a special risk of its own. For the 'fit' may
be succeeded by a period during which the person behaves
like an automaton, when his actions are not under the control of his will, and sometimes quite out of character. It is
possible that some crimes have been committed by persons
in this state, unknowingly.

The 'brain wave', as well as confirming known cases of
epilepsy, sometimes suggests its existence in people who are
not known to have had fits. What is still more remarkable,
an abnormal E.E.G. may be found in the near relatives of
such people. These observations are helping doctors to trace
the cause of epilepsy, which has for long been a mystery.
Almost the only theory which has stood the test of time is
that heredity has something to do with it—not necessarily
that the disorder is inherited, but rather that a constitution
susceptible to it is. This seems borne out by what has just
been said about the 'family' E.E.G.s. One thing is certain,
that ordinary epilepsy is not due to any disease of the brain.
It is due to an occasional failure, under as yet unknown
conditions, of the very complex mechanism which regulates
the energy produced by the cells of the central nervous
system, of which the brain is part. Incidentally, it does not
follow that an epileptic person will have children similarly

afflicted; it has been calculated that the odds against this are over 30–1. Moreover, it is rare for more than one child in such a family to be affected. All the same, as even long odds sometimes come off, sufferers from this disorder might well hesitate to have children.

Although we do not fully understand the nature of the event which, so to speak, 'triggers-off' an epileptic seizure, we know something of what is happening in the brain at the time. Our new helper, the E.E.G., tells that just before and during a fit there are relatively big discharges of electricity from all over the part of the brain known as the 'cortex', followed by electrical 'deadness' which may last for some minutes. (By the way, these phenomena are merely accompaniments of the activity of the nerve-cells; we must firmly reject the notion that the brain works by electricity.) This sequence of activity and quiescence suggests that, in the first phase, the brain-cells, discharging themselves in cascades of energy, stimulate nerve impulses, which in turn excite the muscles to outbursts of undisciplined effort—the typical convulsive movements of the fit. It further suggests that in the second phase, exhaustion of the cells produces the loss of consciousness. If the exhaustion is only partial, not total, this may account for the strangely disordered 'automatic' behaviour which we have already described as happening in some cases.

Generally speaking, there is no likelihood of detecting in advance liability to epileptic attacks unless all the population were subjected to E.E.G. tests. It might be worth while, however, for a person with epilepsy in his family to undergo this test. In any case prevention—in the strict sense of the word—cannot be assured; but epilepsy can readily be controlled, and sufferers enabled to lead reasonably normal and happy lives by the continued use of certain drugs. At one time a number of so-called cures were offered to the public, but their worthlessness may be judged from the fact that their advertisement is now forbidden by law.

PARKINSON'S DISEASE

DOCTORS use the term 'nervous diseases' in a way which is frequently misunderstood by the public. To most people the word 'nervous' has what we might call the strictly psychological meaning: we say that some people are of a nervous disposition, we speak of nervousness, of an attack of nerves, and so on—perfectly legitimate expressions if they are properly applied. In this popular use 'nervous' denotes some quality of temperament, not a state of disease. To a doctor, however, 'nervous' has two distinct meanings. One variety, the so-called 'functional nervous disease', may indeed embrace some of the conditions popularly termed 'nervous', though it goes far beyond mere peculiarities of temperament. But the other variety, 'organic nervous disease', is quite outside the popular meaning and is equally distinct from the 'functional'. It is organic nervous disease which forms a principal part of the branch of medicine called 'neurology'.

We know that the brain communicates with all parts of the body by means of the spinal cord, a kind of 'cable' which lies within a canal enclosed by the backbone. From the spinal cord, at various levels, proceed nerves which run to their particular destinations. These nerves transmit the 'orders' of the brain, and also convey to the brain the 'messages' they receive from the outlying regions. The brain and the spinal cord are collectively known as the 'central nervous system' (C.N.S.), and upon the integrity of this system the functioning of the body primarily depends. The C.N.S., however, is liable to many derangements, and the consequences of these are the 'organic' nervous diseases.

Thus, in a condition known as 'disseminated sclerosis', patches of hardening tissue appear in the spinal cord, the nerve-cells in the affected areas gradually die out, and the parts of the body which were connected to them are cut off from communication with the brain. As it is usually 'motor' areas which are affected, the patient slowly becomes paralysed. In another condition called 'syringomyelia', cavities develop in the substance of the spinal cord. As 'sensory' areas are first affected, a leading symptom is loss of sensation in the corresponding regions of the body, particularly an inability to distinguish heat from cold.

It is impossible to speak accurately of a 'typical' organic nervous disease, for the group is a large one and its members vary widely in their symptoms. They have in common only the feature that there is some physical process of degeneration going on in the central nervous system, usually of unknown or doubtful origin. But a particularly interesting variety may be selected for description. 'Parkinson's Disease' (called so after the nineteenth-century physician who first described it scientifically), is also known as *paralysis agitans*, or, in common speech, 'the shaking palsy'. This malady has been known from ancient times, and little more is known today of its causation than our forefathers knew. With an exception which we shall note later, it rarely arises before the age of 50, and men are affected twice as commonly as women. Essentially, it consists of a stiffening of the muscles accompanied by weakness and trembling, these symptoms coming on very slowly and increasing gradually until the victim becomes quite helpless. It gives rise to a very singular and unmistakable facial expression, the rigidity of the muscles of the face producing a mask-like appearance. The body adopts a stooping posture, with the head and neck sloping forwards, and when the disease is advanced the whole of the trunk moves with the head instead of the latter turning independently. The Parkinsonian patient having difficulty in balancing his body, tends to adopt a peculiar gait, shuffling along in short steps; if he is pushed from behind he keeps going in the endeavour to preserve his balance. The trembling, which comes in time to affect all parts, usually begins with the hand (this is indeed one of the earliest symptoms to be noticed), the fingers acquiring an odd purposeless movement akin to cigarette-rolling. Throughout all this the patient's mind remains unaffected, and he may live for many years.

The cause of Parkinson's Disease is unknown. The only physical change that can be detected in the structure of the body is a degeneration of certain cells in the brain, and presumably it is this that accounts for the symptoms. But what instigates the change we do not know. No treatment yet known can do more than alleviate the distressing symptoms. Certain drugs, chiefly the 'alkaloids' atropine and hyoscine, were formerly used, but nowadays 'synthetic' (artificially manufactured) preparations have to some extent taken their place. A substance called amphetamine, one of the 'pepping-up' drugs said to be used to sustain the morale of certain shock troops in the late war, is also used, but of course none of these drugs may be taken except under medical supervision. Recently it has been suggested that Parkinsonism may actually be cured by an operation on the brain, and, indeed, a number of such operations have been performed. But we have not yet nearly sufficient experience to know positively what lasting benefit may be expected or what disadvantages may attend this delicate procedure.

There is an exception to the rule that Parkinsonism is a disease of later life, known as 'post-encephalitic Parkinsonism'. During and after the First World War an epidemic ran through the world of what appeared to be an entirely new disease, named *encephalitis lethargica* ('sleepy sickness'), essentially an inflammation of the brain, apparently due to a virus. After running for some years this epidemic subsided rapidly and the disease is now seldom heard of. The point of interest for our present purpose is that *encephalitis lethargica* usually attacked young people, and was frequently followed by a condition known as 'post-encephalitic Parkinsonism', with symptoms exceedingly like those of the familiar Parkinson's Disease.

BLINDNESS

WHEN we speak of the 'mind's eye' we are speaking physiologically more truly than we realize, for it is really the brain that does the 'seeing'. The eye is but the instrument by which the range of electro-magnetic vibrations we call 'light' are changed into a form capable of stimulating the visual centre of the brain, and so producing certain sensations. Out of these sensations the mind creates the patterns which we call sight. It is conceivable that some day an electronic device may be invented to make an artificial eye to function as an artificial limb does, but so fantastic a possibility is now far from realization. Such a device, in any case, would serve only the function of the eye, and could not produce sight unless it were connected with that irreplaceable organ of perception which resides in the depths of the brain.

In the older books on popular physiology the eye used to be regarded as merely an optical instrument, usually compared with a camera. This was an over-simplification. In its basic construction the eye is, up to a point, analogous to any optical system which is capable of forming a 'real' image; but beyond that point other physical and chemical phenomena begin to operate. The eye consists, as we know, of a globe divided vertically into two chambers, a small one in front, a much larger one behind. In the front chamber is the 'lens', an object exactly like a magnifying-glass but capable of altering its curvature and hence its focal length, and fitted with a contracting diaphragm (iris) just like the similarly named component of a camera. The lens and iris are protected by a transparent shield, the 'cornea', which covers them in front. The front chamber is filled with a fluid, the 'aqueous humour'. The back chamber is filled with a kind of jelly called the 'vitreous humour'. This series of re-fractive media—the cornea, lens, aqueous and vitreous humours—go to make an 'achromatic' system, just like the several lenses of different kinds of glass which compose a high-grade optical instrument.

Right at the back of the rear compartment, opposite and farthest from the lens, is the 'retina', and it is at this point that our optical system ends. You see how it works—the lens, whose aperture is controlled by the iris according to the intensity of the illumination, brings to a focus rays of light emitted by or reflected from external objects. The varying distances of objects are compensated for by varying the curvature of the lens, not, as in ordinary optical instruments, by mov-ing the lens back and forth (the alteration of lens-curvature is brought about by the action of a surrounding muscle). The focused image is cast on the retina, inverted and much smaller than the object it pictures, just as in a camera.

Now begins the process of conveying the image to the brain, and this resembles television-camera practice rather than ordinary photography. For the retina is not a solid screen of homogeneous composition; it consists of layers of highly specialized cells, and each point of the image cast upon it is dealt with separately by the cells in whose area it happens to fall. The image is really being decomposed, an-alysed, or broken-up just as optical images are in television cameras or in half-tone processes of reproduction; it now consists of a mosaic of infinitesimally small pieces which, taken as a whole, compose an apparently continuous pattern. (There is just one point which should be made clear—in the building up of the visual image there is nothing equivalent to the 'scanning' process of television, the entire image is dealt with simultaneously by the retinal layers of cells.)

But still we have not got vision. We have only projected the image of external objects on to a sensitive screen. The next step is for each of the multitude of elements composing the screen to deal with its particular bit of the image, and this involves an exceedingly complicated physico-chemical process. Put very briefly, when light falls on the retina a chemical change takes place which has the effect of generating minute electric currents (this statement must not be taken too literally; it is made by way of analogy with familiar things). These currents ultimately create a series of impulses in the 'optic nerve' which conveys them to the brain. This nerve has somewhat the function of the 'co-axial cable' of television, and it carries multi-currents of differing phase. (We must not regard this metaphor as an actual explanation of what is taking place, it is simply the nearest we can get to the facts without employing unintelligibly technical language.) There I am afraid we must leave it; the action of the parts of the brain described as the 'visuo-sensory' and 'visuo-psychic' areas (the true residence of the sense of sight) is much too complicated for anyone but a specialist to understand.

Now it will be evident from what we have said that there is plenty of room for things to go wrong at any stage of the process of vision. Some part of the brain concerned with the reception or the interpretation of the nerve-impulses may be absent or non-functioning. The optic nerve may be interrupted by injury or disease. The retina may be damaged. The transparent parts of the eye, the lens or the cornea, may become opaque. If any of these conditions exist, blindness follows. Some of them may be congenital in that an essential part may have failed to develop before birth, and this usually cannot be made good. Blindness can result from various forms of inflammation of the eye which destroy its tissues. Some of these inflammations are due to local infections, of which one can be conveyed to a child at the moment of birth because the mother suffers from a venereal disease (see p. 19). Certain poisons, some general diseases, and destructive local injuries of many kinds can cause blindness. Among the less frequent causes is severe haemorrhage in any part of the body, for great loss of blood, such as follows internal bleeding, can cause blindness because the vital tissues of the eye are not adequately nourished.

But it is our purpose to speak rather of those conditions wherein there is hope for the restoration of sight, and happily their number is growing. The first kind of blindness to be overcome was that caused by 'cataract'. In this, which afflicts chiefly persons past middle-age (though there are occasional exceptions, and even some congenital cases, and a form known as 'traumatic' cataract—a result of injury— can attack persons at any age), the lens becomes opaque and no light can enter the eye. The radical cure in such cases is to remove the lens, making good its loss by fitting the patient with extra-strong spectacles. A recent development of the operation provides for the insertion of an artificial 'plastic' lens in place of the natural lens when the latter has been extracted. Then there is 'corneal opacity', which commonly follows some injury (such as burning, splashing with acid, or ulceration) to the cornea (the transparent part of the eyeball in front of the lens). Recently, in a number of cases, the resultant blindness has been cured by cutting a piece out of the opaque cornea and grafting in a piece of transparent tissue taken from another eye, thus making, as it were, a window through which light can pass to the lens.

'Glaucoma' is a serious condition responsible for many cases of blindness. In this the fluid contents of the eye increase in bulk, and exert undue pressure over the whole interior of the eyeball, including of course the retina, seriously deranging its delicate mechanism. The patient's field of view gradually shrinks, he sees the world as if he were looking through a decreasing aperture, till finally all vision is lost. As the maleficent condition is the abnormal internal tension of the eyeball, the remedy is to relieve this, if possible. This may be done by draining off some of the fluid contents, or by assisting the natural process of drainage. There are medical methods of attempting this, but until quite recently various surgical operations were preferred, in particular the one called 'trephining'. It has lately been suggested, however, that a 'hormone' called 'ACTH' for short (its proper name is too unwieldy for everyday use) is efficacious in treatment. Intensive research is proceeding along this line.

As we have just mentioned the possibility of the medical treatment of threatening blindness this is the appropriate place to describe another kind of disaster—the complete shutting off of the circulation of the retina through blockage of its blood-vessels by a clot. This condition, known as 'retinal thrombosis', causes sudden and total blindness, and was formerly regarded as irremediable. But it is now possible, if immediate action be taken, to dissolve the clot by means of 'anticoagulant' drugs (see p. 65). Unfortunately, it seldom happens that this treatment can be applied before irreparable injury has been done to the retina through the failure of its circulation.

One of the most spectacular advances in our counter-attack against threats to sight is the operative treatment of 'detachment of the retina'. In this condition, once thought practically hopeless, the layers at the back of the eye separate and peel off so that the functioning of the retina is impaired.

This condition can occur as a result of injury or disease, or perhaps of predisposition. Only a few years ago the most we could do for the victim was to keep him lying flat on his back for many months in the hope that the detached tissue would settle down in position again, which it rarely did. But now it has been discovered that this detachment is usually preceded by a hole or tear in the retina, and an operation to repair this perforation by means of an electro-cautery has been devised. In a high proportion of cases permanent replacement and full restoration of vision follow.

It is estimated that there are not less than 100,000 blind persons in Great Britain alone. Sad as it is to contemplate the number of people who are shut out from the world of sight, their total would be far greater were it not for the progress of medical science. Perhaps even among the 100,000 there are some who may yet live literally to see further advances which will lighten their darkness.

DEAFNESS

IT is curious and dismaying that there is a less sympathetic attitude towards loss of hearing than towards loss of sight. The difficulties of the blind evoke universal understanding and compassion, but the handicaps of the deaf too often provoke only a feeling of irritation. This is quite illogical and very wrong. In many respects the deaf are more completely isolated from human fellowship than the blind, and they are acutely sensitive of their lack. Although they have the gift of sight, it is not an unmixed blessing, for it enables them to see impatience in the faces of those whom their infirmity exasperates. We all have some experience of sightlessness—in the dark all alike are blind—but there is in our normal lives no parallel to deafness, which obliterates alike music, the voices of friends, the pleasant sounds of nature.

The organs of hearing are of very complicated and delicate structure, even more complicated and delicate, in some ways, than the eye. The part that we see is only a funnel for the collection and concentration of sound-waves, something like the mouthpiece of a telephone. What we call the ear—the fleshy fold that projects from the side of the head—is properly the 'auricle'. Leading from this inwards is the 'external auditory meatus', a short passage which is closed at its inner end by the eardrum, or 'tympanic membrane'. Sound-waves proceeding through the meatus cause this membrane to vibrate—again as happens in the telephone, in which also there is a vibrating 'diaphragm'. But when we come to the end of the visible parts of the ear, we out-distance our telephone analogy and enter a very compli-cated field of anatomy and physiology.

Immediately behind the eardrum are the 'ossicles', a flexible chain of three very small bones of peculiar shape, called respectively, the 'malleus', 'incus', and 'stapes'—names that indicate their shapes. The ossicles are situated in a chamber known as the 'tympanic cavity' or 'middle ear', and they stretch right across it from the eardrum in its outer wall to the opposite wall on the inside. Beyond this wall is the 'internal ear'. Both the middle ear and the internal ear are imbedded in the bones of the skull—to one of these bones, known as the 'mastoid process', we shall have further occasion to refer. The middle ear communicates with the back of the throat through a passage called the 'Eustachian tube', which has the function of equalizing the air-pressure on both sides of the eardrum. This passage also will call for our further notice.

We said that the ossicles span the width of the tympanic cavity. The innermost one, the 'stapes', is formed like a stirrup. That part of it which corresponds to the stirrup's foot-plate fits exactly in an oval opening on the inside wall of the cavity. This window-like opening, the *fenestra vesti-buli*, is covered with a thin membrane like a miniature drum. We have now reached the 'labyrinth', the beginning of the internal ear, the true organ of hearing. The construction of this labyrinth is, as the name implies, exceedingly complex, and only a very simplified account of it can be given here. There are in fact two concentric labyrinths, an osseous (bony) one enclosing a membranous inner organ. The principal part of the osseous labyrinth consists of a tube made of bone, coiled spirally, which, from its resemblance to a snail-shell, is known as the 'cochlea'. This tube is filled with a fluid called 'perilymph', and within it floats, so to speak, the membranous labyrinth which in turn is filled with 'endolymph'. But here we also find a most important structure named, after its discoverer, the 'organ of Corti'. The function of the organ of Corti is comparable with that of the retina of the eye (see p. 116), in that each is responsible for transmuting external physical stimuli into nerve impulses able to reach the brain. In the ear this sensitive organ, which may be regarded as an extension of the auditory nerve, contains many thousands of minute fibres called 'hair cells', and it is by the stimulation of these cells that the auditory nerve is made to convey to the hearing centre of the brain the sensations which we recognize as 'sounds'.

The final stages of hearing are, like the final stages of seeing, not fully understood, but up to this last perceptive operation the process is something like this. Sound-waves, propagated in the air from any source capable of setting up the necessary vibrations, travel through the external auditory meatus until they impinge on the tympanum, and cause it to vibrate. At the back of the tympanum is the chain of ossicles which serves the double purpose of 'damping' the vibrations of the tympanic membrane (preventing its uncontrolled movement back and forth) and of transmitting these vibrations first to the vestibule of the inner ear, and then to the cochlea and the organ of Corti. It is necessary here to mention that the inner ear also contains very important structures known as the 'semicircular canals'; these are a kind of spirit-level which preserve our bodily equilibrium, and without which we should not know if we were lying down or standing up—indeed, we should not be able to balance ourselves in an erect posture. But the semicircular canals, although highly important and interesting, have nothing to do with the faculty of hearing.

There is obviously plenty of room for something to go wrong with the ear, which is subject to many diseases, some resulting in total or partial deafness. Those unfortunate people who are born deaf are also often dumb, not necessarily because they are wanting the organs of speech, or because the 'speech centre' of the brain is defective, but simply because, never having heard sounds, they have never learned to imitate them. It is quite possible to teach such deaf-mutes to speak by special methods of training. The so-called 'congenital' deafness is due to a defect of the hearing centre of the brain, or of the auditory nerve, or of an essential part of the internal ear. These defects are irremediable, and must cause lifelong deafness.

Among the number of general diseases which can spread inflammation to the ear and, by destroying parts of it, cause deafness, are some infections especially common in children, such as mumps, scarlet fever, measles, and meningitis. Certain other diseases such as tuberculosis, syphilis, and even arthritis may cause deafness in varying degree. Broadly speaking, anything which produces inflammation of the middle or inner parts of the ear may result in deafness. Thus, a more or less temporary deafness is often caused by catarrh, for as the middle cavity of the ear communicates with the back of the throat through the Eustachian tube, it is easy for catarrh in the nose or throat to extend up these tubes into the ear. A serious form of inflammation is that known as 'otitis media', in which severe suppuration of the middle ear may set up such pressure as to make the eardrum bulge outwards and burst. Sometimes the drum has to be deliberately pierced by the surgeon to prevent this; but this 'perforation' of the eardrum—or even its complete removal —does not necessarily produce total deafness, since the vibrations of sound-waves may still be conveyed through the ossicles. Even the loss of the ossicles can leave the patient with some degree of hearing, provided that the inner ear is intact. Otitis media occurs in both acute and chronic forms, the latter often subsequent to the former. By more effective treatment of the acute form, we have reduced the incidence of chronic otitis media, which used to be very common.

Another kind of ear inflammation is 'mastoiditis', or 'mastoid disease' as it is often called. This is not primarily an ear disease, but is an inflammation of one of the bones of the skull—the 'mastoid process'—in which part of the ear is embedded. Usually the mastoid becomes inflamed because infection has spread to it from a diseased middle ear; and so we nearly always have preliminary signs of trouble in the ear itself. Mastoiditis is an extremely serious condition, which, neglected, may have many and dire consequences— even death, either from meningitis (see p. 105) or from general blood-poisoning (*septicaemia*). In one form of operation for mastoid disease, an opening in the skull is made, behind the auricle, to drain off the pus which has filled the honeycomb-like structure of the mastoid. In another operation (the so-called 'radical') a great deal of bone has to be cut away, leaving a large cavity which involves both the mastoid and the middle ear. But modern methods of treating local infections by the use of sulphonamides and antibiotics have reduced the need for these drastic procedures.

There is another and gradual form of deafness caused by what is called 'otosclerosis'. This is often the origin of the proverbial 'hardness of hearing' of elderly people, but it may affect quite young men and women. We saw how the footplate of the 'stapes' was inserted in the *fenestra vestibuli*. It normally has some freedom of movement, but in otosclerosis it becomes fixed. Until quite recently no treatment was effective, but there has now been devised an exceedingly delicate operation called 'fenestration' which has given very good results.

Once upon a time a famous doctor said, 'There are two forms of deafness: one is caused by wax and is curable; the other is not caused by wax and is incurable.' There is no need to hold so pessimistic an opinion nowadays. Most forms of deafness can be alleviated, some even cured. Many of the deaf for whom medicine or surgery can do nothing, can be helped by modern electronic devices which amplify sounds. Some of these devices, based on 'bone-conduction', convey the sound-waves not through the auricle, but through the bones of the skull straight to the inner ear. There the organ of Corti, stimulated by these vibrations, translates them into the same kind of impulses as it would normally-conveyed sound-waves. The ultimate effect is therefore that of sound.

Sudden deafness, especially in one ear only, is usually caused by a plug of hardened wax blocking the meatus. The walls of the meatus secrete a soft wax which normally covers them, probably to trap small foreign bodies and prevent their reaching the drum. Excessive wax formation blocks the orifice or coats the surface of the drum. It is not safe to use domestic remedies for removing the wax. If a doctor syringes the ear, the hearing will be immediately restored.

FRACTURES

MORE than once when, making sympathetic inquiry after the victim of an accident, I have asked, 'Were any bones broken?' I have received the answer, 'Oh no—the doctor said Johnny had only *fractured* his arm (leg, skull, ribs, collarbone, backbone).' From this I infer that in some people's minds there is a distinction between a fracture and a break. But in fact, in the surgery as in the dictionary, the two words are synonymous.

Bones are of various shape, according to their purpose. Some are long like the thigh-bone, some flat like the shoulder-blade, some curved like the ribs, some short cylinders like those of the hands and feet, some more or less cubical like the bones of the spine, some of irregular shape like the skull and the pelvis. Whatever their shape, size, or position any of them can get broken, in spite of the fact that bone is about twice as strong as seasoned oak-wood.

Fractures are of different kinds. There is the simple or 'closed' fracture, in which a bone is snapped asunder like a dry twig but without wounding the surrounding parts. There is the compound or 'open' fracture in which not only is the bone broken but soft parts also are injured, allowing ingress of foreign matter from without. There is a type of fracture sometimes described as 'complicated' in which the broken bone injures an internal organ without causing an opening to the exterior. There is the 'comminuted' fracture in which the bone is shattered into several pieces; and there is the 'greenstick' fracture (the only one which may justify the popular error that a fracture is not a break) in which the bone is not cleanly broken asunder but is partly broken and partly bent as a piece of soft timber might be if we tried to snap it. There are sub-varieties of these different kinds of fractures, classified according to their origin and the complications they cause. I shall mention only one here—the 'impacted' fracture in which the parts of the broken bone are driven firmly into one another by the force of the accident.

There is a point about fractures which is sometimes overlooked. Bones, as well as supporting our bodies and acting as a safe-guarding framework for some of our organs, must serve as anchorages for our muscles, the contraction and expansion of which causes our limbs to move. There must therefore be at times a considerable 'pull' from the muscles, which the natural rigidity of the bones resists. But if a bone is broken, this pull tends to displace the broken ends and may even cause them to overlap. When this has happened, the broken ends must, before the bone can be 'set', be replaced in contact with each other in their proper position, a manœuvre called 'reduction'.

How is it that a bone, once broken, can repair itself? We must remember that bone is not a dead substance but a living tissue, just as flesh is. We all know how a flesh wound heals (when we come to think of it the flesh has really been 'broken', although we speak of it as cut or torn); and the healing of bone begins in the same way. In both cases, in a process akin to sock-darning, a new material called 'granulation tissue' bridges the gap; and this later turns into fibrous tissue, which is tougher stuff. In the case of a wound of the soft parts of the body, the new tissue then 'skins over', and in due course we say the wound has healed—usually leaving a scar to mark its place. But there is a very important difference in the healing of bone. Whereas with the soft parts of the body all that is needed is so to speak to fill up the hole, with bone we may have to make a repair strong enough to take a very heavy load. It would not suffice to repair a broken bone with fibrous tissue, for this would be like trying to repair broken metal with glue. Glue is all very well for woodwork, but for metal we must solder or braze.

Up to the stage of forming fibrous tissue, therefore, the healing of flesh and bone follows an identical course; but at this point in healing broken bone, when the pieces of bone are merely stuck together so that the joint would break again if any pressure were put on it, the new tissue is saturated with lime (the chief constituent of all bone) till eventually it becomes a solid mass surrounding the fracture. This mass, at first chalklike, gradually hardens into real bone, the entire process of repair usually taking upwards of six weeks. The knob of material which surrounds a healing fracture is called 'callus': when it is quite soft, it is called 'ensheathing' callus; when chalky, 'calcified' callus; when bony, 'permanent' callus. The final appearance resembles what a plumber calls a 'wiped joint' in piping.

The repair of fractures is a natural process, which we can assist only by providing the right conditions. The broken ends of bone must be brought into close contact in their proper position, and kept there until permanent callus has formed. With a straight-forward fracture this is done by splinting the injured parts (first having replaced them in their proper position, if necessary). Splints are of course applied outside a limb. Sometimes, as in fractures of the spine, the injured part is encased in plaster of Paris which sets solid around it. But some bones, and some kinds of fractures, are not amenable to this relatively simple treatment. The broken ends will not remain in position unless they are subjected to 'continuous traction'. This is generally accomplished by hanging a weight on to the end of a limb by means of cords running over pulleys (a device often employed for fractured thighs). Sometimes a bone is so badly shattered that, to keep the broken bits in position, it is necessary to wire them together, or even to use metal side-plates with bolts which screw into the bone. In one case, that of fractures of the neck of the femur (the upper end of the thighbone where it is jointed into the hip), the broken pieces are often actually nailed together by a long metal spike driven through them. This procedure, which marks an important advance in the treatment of fractures, enables many people to walk soon after their accident who would formerly have been crippled for life. All these methods may be regarded as a kind of internal splinting, the 'splints' being applied to the bone itself instead of to the outside of the limb (though the latter must be protected as well for a time). Another method, where pegs of bone or other substances are used which later become absorbed, we may regard as intermediate between internal splinting and natural repair.

There is still the treatment of impacted fractures and compound fractures to consider. Their treatment follows the usual lines, but with impacted fractures, before the bones can be replaced in their proper position, the two pieces of bone which have been 'telescoped' may need to be drawn apart. This can be difficult to do, for sometimes they have been driven together very firmly indeed, and often there is a lot of splintering of bone all around. We may have deliberately to turn a naturally 'closed' or simple fracture into an 'open' or compound one before we can treat it. With certain kinds of impacted fractures, however, it assists the process of repair to leave them untouched. With an open fracture the wound as well must be treated. Sometimes the fracture itself has made the wound, the sharp end of a broken bone piercing the flesh, sometimes the injury is from without, involving bone and flesh; but in either case the wound must be cleaned up and kept free from infection so that it heals as the bone heals.

In spite of everything we can do it occasionally happens that a broken bone just will not 'knit'. The ends stick together after a fashion, but the fashion is that which plumbers call a 'dry joint'. The joint is made only by 'fibrous union', for no calcified callus has formed and the broken ends are not truly united. As these fibrous unions are often fairly strong, the part may be usable to a moderate extent, and with some bones the need for absolute repair is not so important as with others. But failure to achieve a proper bony union is generally considered an unsatisfactory result.

STRAINS, SPRAINS, AND DISLOCATIONS

STRICTLY speaking, the word 'strain' has no special medical significance. It means what it usually does in everyday speech; that is to say, a condition in which something has been put on the stretch. It follows that any part of the body which has been so treated—muscles, ligaments, tendons, or the like—may be described as 'strained'. It does not follow that any actual injury has resulted, any more than would result to a piece of elastic that was stretched. But just as it is possible to overstretch elastic so that it doesn't 'go back' when released, so we can overstretch our muscle or whatever it is. There is this important difference, that the muscle &c., if rested, can recover 'tone', whereas the elastic cannot. It is not necessarily violent effort which produces a strain, though of course it is the most likely cause; relatively slight but continued efforts in unnatural postures (as in some games) can also produce it. It is worthy of note that when we walk upright about 150 muscles are concerned with the simple task of keeping the back straight, so it is not surprising that anything which upsets muscle-balance can strain something or other—the really surprising thing is how difficult it is normally to upset that balance. Provided that no muscle, ligament, tendon, or what not has been torn, the strain need give no serious trouble. To ensure that the strained part is rested we sometimes strap it up with sticking-plaster—adequate treatment for a simple strain.

Now we will consider a 'sprain', which is often confused with strain, not unnaturally since the two are closely associated. A strain can exist without causing a sprain, but the occurrence of a sprain presupposes a condition of temporary and violent strain. A sprain always occurs at joints, whereas a strain can affect these or other ('non-articular') parts of the body.

Joints, or 'articulations', consist of the ends of bones fitted together so that they can move after the fashion of hinges, ball-and-sockets, &c. To be exact these freely movable junctions such as ankle, wrist, knee, or elbow, should be called 'synovial joints'—there are other kinds which do not move freely, but it is only synovial joints that we shall now consider. In joints of this kind the ends of the bones are covered with a smooth layer of 'cartilage', and between them is a cavity containing a small quantity of 'synovial fluid' (which is prevented from running out by being enclosed within a 'capsule'). The bones are bound together by strong ligaments which, while allowing the movement proper to the joint, normally prevent its being broken apart. There is a lot more anatomical detail to joints than this simple account implies, but that is all we need to know for our present purpose.

A sprain occurs when a joint has been violently strained, usually by wrenching or twisting, and when its binding ligaments have been torn. This injury is followed by a swelling, caused by bleeding of torn tissues beneath the skin, and sometimes also by an escape of the synovial fluid. This is a very painful affair which definitely puts the joint out of action. Treatment resembles that for a strain up to a point, that is, we must rest the affected part; no attempt must be made to use the joint until all the swelling has gone. But the greater severity of the condition calls for additional remedies. As the origin of the sprain was the over-stretching of the ligaments, bandaging is necessary to take the strain off the torn tissues. This is done by strapping up the joint with sticking-plaster when it is in a position where there is no 'pull' on the ligaments. After the swelling has subsided, a little massage and some gentle movement is helpful. The effects of a severe sprain may last for weeks, and if it is neglected or improperly treated, it can give rise to trouble in after life.

We have spoken of strains, which may or may not involve joints; and of sprains which always involve joints, but do not affect the bones. Now we must consider dislocations, which are displacements of the bones of a joint. As explained above, these bones are normally bound together by very strong ligaments, so that no ordinary force can separate them. But if the ligaments are very much over-stretched and torn, and the force which has done this continues to be applied to the joint, the bones may be drawn or 'levered' apart—pulled out of their sockets—and displaced from their proper positions. Sometimes the bones are separated only momentarily and 'snap' back again; but often the displacement is complete, and the joint remains dislocated until the bones are skilfully replaced in position. Much more extensive injury may follow dislocation than the simple displacement of the bones—there may be severe damage to 'soft tissues' as well. Again, dislocation may accompany fractures or other injuries; the co-existence of a fracture and a dislocation presents the surgeon with a difficult problem. But an uncomplicated dislocation is fairly simple to deal with, for example, expert manipulation can 'put back' a dislocated shoulder with apparent ease. In other cases—many of them, like some dislocations of the thumb, seemingly straight-forward—appearances are deceptive; internal injuries, which cannot be put right by any external handling, necessitate an operation. So it is not wise to be too enthusiastic in first-aid. It is better to play for safety, remembering that no harm can ever be done by the temporary immobilization of joint or limb, whereas very great harm may follow well-meaning but injudicious attempts to anticipate the doctor.

A rather curious kind of 'joint' injury has received a good deal of notice of late years, the so-called 'slipped disk'. The 'joints' involved, however—those between the spinal vertebrae—are not ordinarily regarded as such. The spine consists of a column of bones each one of which is, roughly speaking, shaped like a short hollow cylinder—they are as it were 'threaded' on the spinal cord. But these bones are not in actual contact with one another, for between each is a pad of cartilage known as an 'intervertebral disk'. Certain kinds of injury (even very slight ones such as particular strains) can damage a disk, which may thus be crushed or broken in one or several places. As a result the disk, or part of it, may be pushed out of its normal position between the vertebrae, and the adjacent bones to some extent displaced. If the 'slipped disk' is low down in the back, sciatica may follow as a result of pressure on the nerve; if it is higher up, the victim may suffer a kind of neuritis of the arm. Many hitherto unaccountable pains in the back and limbs have been traced to these 'disk lesions'. It is quite a serious condition: often patients have to wear a rigid 'corset' or a plaster jacket for a time; sometimes cure is impossible without a surgical operation.

HERNIA (*RUPTURE*)

As often happens, the popular term for this condition is both more graphic and more descriptive than the technical. For 'rupture' describes the initial happening, and 'hernia' the development.

The trunk of the human body is divided transversely into two compartments. The upper, the thorax, contains the heart and lungs; the lower compartment, the abdomen, contains a number of other organs very closely packed together. It is this second compartment which is our concern now. Let us first think of the abdomen as if it were an empty cavity. It is roofed in by the diaphragm, which divides it from the thorax (just as the ceiling of one room is the floor of the one above); its lower part rests on the pelvis as on a foundation; its front and sides consist of muscles; its back, muscled too, contains the lower and middle part of the spine which we can regard as a great column supporting the whole. The front and sides of the abdomen, themselves unsupported, consist of 'soft tissues', and they retain their proper shape only because these tissues are (or should be) strong muscles with the power of contracting to bind the whole together. The inside wall of the cavity is lined with a membrane called the peritoneum.

Now let us look at the abdomen when it is filled, as it is in nature. The organs of digestion are the main contents, and notably the intestines. These 'tubes' are approximately between twenty and thirty feet long and from one to three inches in diameter. To coil away into the space between the diaphragm and the pelvis not only this length of piping, but several other sizeable organs, calls for tight packing; and the intestines are, through their bulk and weight, exerting constant internal pressure on the abdominal wall, much as are the contents of an over-full bag. Generally speaking, the

muscles of the abdominal wall are well calculated to resist
this pressure, but the wall has certain weak places, notably
at the navel and at the groin. It is at the groin that rupture
most commonly occurs, when, for some reason, there is an
increase of the strain on the muscles of the abdominal wall
—it may be, for example, that a person has made some unusually heavy effort of lifting. The extra strain overcomes
the resistance of the wall at the weakest spot (just as the
attempt to pack more stuff into an already full bag causes
a weak seam to give way), and a 'sac' is formed there. This
sac at first is just a depression in the lining of the abdominal
cavity, the peritoneum. But behind this depression is a loop
of intestine pushing away at the weak place, deepening the
depression till it becomes a definite pouch visible and palp-
able as a swelling in the groin. This swelling, the hernial sac,
consists of all the layers of the abdominal wall from the
peritoneum on the inside to the skin on the outside, with a
loop of intestine filling it.

There are several varieties of rupture. Contrary to the
popular belief, either sex can be affected, though different
forms of rupture are more usual in one than the other. Some
persons are particularly prone to become ruptured because
their abdominal walls are congenitally weaker at the
normally weak places. But wherever a rupture is, and however it is caused, its fundamental feature is the hernial sac
and the loop of intestine protruding into it. It may seem that
this is after all no very great matter, but in fact the condition
is one that must be dealt with as quickly as possible. In the
first place, once a rupture is established, any physical effort
is likely to aggravate it—the sac stretches and more intestine
pushes its way into it. Then it must be remembered that
the intestine is not a passive structure; it is behaving as an
active part of the digestive system through which solids and
liquids are passing all the time. Now, should the neck of the

sac constrict so that the loop becomes 'nipped' and its contents cannot move one way or the other, we shall have the condition called strangulated hernia. This is followed by intestinal obstruction, one of the most serious emergencies doctors have to deal with. Moreover, the nipped loop may have its blood-circulation impeded; it may become gangrenous and then only immediate operation can save the patient's life.

At one time the only means used to relieve ordinary ruptures was the wearing of a truss. This is a kind of open belt, usually made of a semi-rigid springy material, with a padded metal band at the end (or two pads for 'double rupture'), worn so as to press on the swelling and keep the loop of intestine from coming down into the hernial sac. But trusses do not cure rupture, they only make it possible for persons wearing them to engage in some physical activities which otherwise would be dangerous. The only means of curing the condition is to replace the loop of intestine permanently inside the abdomen and to obliterate the hernial sac. This is what is done in the so-called radical operation. After the sac has been opened and the intestinal loop returned to where it belongs, the now empty sac is cut off, and the hole remaining in the abdominal wall is repaired layer by layer by the usual surgical methods. After this operation the patient may be said to be better than ever, for, as the weak place in the abdominal wall has been strengthened, the liability to rupture at that spot is practically abolished.

HERPES ZOSTER

THIS disease, better known as 'shingles', is of interest on account of its cause. The popular name has no connexion with Brighton beach or with American roofing material; it

is a corruption of the medical word *cingulus* which is itself
bad Latin (as, I am sorry to say, much medical terminology
is), based on the classical *cingulum* = a girdle. The less
familiar name, 'herpes zoster', is reasonably good Greek,
the second word also meaning 'girdle' and the first being
derived from an expression meaning 'to creep'—hence, by
an extension of metaphor, something serpentine.

A developed case shows a line of little blisters running
round the body at the level of the ribs. This apparent line
consists of a number of groups of these 'blebs' or 'vesicles'.
There is a baseless superstition that, if the line completely
encircles the body, the patient will die; actually the 'girdle'
hardly ever is complete, for reasons which will soon appear.

The earliest noticeable symptom is pain in the place
where the line of vesicles will break out later. This pain increases greatly as the disease progresses till, by the time the
vesicular eruption is well developed, it is very severe indeed.
After some time—which may run into weeks—the eruption
subsides, usually leaving scars where it has been. Occasionally the adjacent muscles may be paralysed to some extent,
and this paralysis can be permanent.

Although the region most commonly affected is that
round the ribs, herpes (not then termed 'zoster') can attack
any part of the body. If the face is affected—as often happens—the symptoms are similar, except that the pain may
be still more intense and a neuralgia may ensue which per-
sists after the eruption has subsided. Paralysis of some of the
facial muscles is quite likely, and occasionally the eruption
reaches the neighbourhood of the eye, starting infection
which may cause loss of sight.

Herpes has every appearance of being a disease of the
skin; but in fact it is a nerve infection. It is due to a virus
which, because it has a particular affinity for nerve-tissue,
is termed neurotropic. This virus attacks a 'ganglion', or

nerve-junction, in the spinal cord, where it sets up an acute inflammation. The inflammation spreads along the course of the nerves which lead from the ganglion to the skin, hence the eruption always follows the 'distribution' of a nerve. As we might expect, facial herpes arises when the Gasserian ganglion is attacked by the virus (see p. 141).

The very much more serious 'poliomyelitis' (see p. 25) is likewise caused by the infection of the spinal nerves through a virus, but, apart from this similarity in the method of causation, there is no connexion between the two. There does, however, appear to be some connexion between herpes and 'chicken-pox' (see p. 32), though its precise nature has not yet been made out. Since, in a number of cases, persons have developed the one disease shortly after being in contact with a patient suffering from the other, some doctors believe that both diseases are due to the same virus, or at least to slightly differing varieties.

Unfortunately there is as yet no specific remedy for herpes, though it is hoped that one of the newest antibiotics may provide it. Meanwhile, the treatment is to soothe the pain by means of various drugs, and to keep the vesicles clean, so that when they break they do not present an opportunity for other germs to enter the body. And, bearing in mind the mysterious relationship between herpes and chicken-pox, we should as far as possible protect ourselves from contact with sufferers from either—especially as having had chicken-pox does not confer protection against herpes, or vice versa.

TRIGEMINAL NEURALGIA
(*TIC DOULOUREUX*)

'There was a young fellow of Deal who said "although pain isn't real, when I sit on a pin and it punctures my skin,

I dislike what I fancy I feel".' This limerick irresistibly comes to the mind when we are told that we do not feel pain in that part of the body where it seems to arise—we feel it in the brain. When the pin punctured the skin it stimulated certain nerve-endings, and this eventually produced a purely mental consciousness of sensation. But it is quite untrue to say that 'pain' does not exist outside the imagination. 'There was never yet philosopher that could endure the toothache patiently', and pain is a reality (that is, as much a reality as any other mental experience). It is also a necessity of life, nature's warning of trouble, and if we lacked it we should undergo various destructive processes without knowing in time to take action. We cannot have things both ways—the nerve-mechanism which makes a corn on the foot so uncomfortable a possession is the same as that which prompts us to drop the hot poker that otherwise would burn our fingers off.

Pain is, of course, one of the sensations which we experience through the sense of 'feeling'. The other senses— sight, hearing, smell, and taste—are localized in particular organs, whereas feeling (touch) appears to be diffused generally throughout the body. Strictly, feeling is not so universal in our frames, which have many quite insensitive areas, and others of varying sensory capacity. Feeling is really quite as specific a sense as any of the other four, and like them it depends on 'end-receptors'. Scattered profusely over the body are certain minute organs of differing constructions whose special function it is to 'pick up' sensations —indeed, these receptors are so intensely specialized that particular groups of them do only particular jobs. Thus, there are some which pick up the sensation of pressure, others that of heat or cold, and others that of pain—in short, all the sensations which go to make up the general sense of 'feeling'. But although the receptor organs are differentiated, their functioning is similar in that each passes on to the brain the sensation appropriate to it. Usually when the brain receives the message, it orders some action designed to deal with the situation it has been warned of—for example, the order to drop the hot poker. But of course not all sensations arise from causes external to the body, and there are many varieties of pain which rouse no such automatic or semi-automatic response.

There is one kind of pain so excruciating that our forefathers called it *tic douloureux*, 'the sorrowful spasm'. Nowadays it is customary to call it 'trigeminal neuralgia'. The word 'neuralgia' does not indicate that the neuralgic pain people often suffer from bears any resemblance to this affliction. The pain affects the face, and is so acute that some victims of this malady have in the past put an end to their lives rather than endure it. The agonizing paroxysms start without the slightest warning, and when they have temporarily subsided, the sufferer is terrified by the possibility of their return. It seems that a very slight cause may provoke them, washing the face, eating, even talking. The acute agony is followed by less severe but more lasting pain, and in bad cases, which have received no treatment, the victim's life is made up of these alternating experiences. It is unusual for persons below middle age to be sufferers, and women are more commonly affected than men.

The actual cause of trigeminal neuralgia is unknown. But the mechanism of the pain is easy to understand. The muscles responsible for those movements of the mouth and jaws which enable us to chew and swallow our food are, like all such muscles, controlled by nerves. The particular nerve which interests us is called the 'fifth' or 'trigeminal' (the latter name because it is divided into three branches), and, like all nerves, it has both motor and sensory functions—that is to say, it transmits 'orders' from the brain to the muscles, and it also conducts to the brain 'messages' which it has picked up from the area which it serves. Anything which irritates it is capable of imparting a more or less painful stimulus. As we all know, decaying teeth can give rise to very painful stimulation of the nerve, as can any kind of local inflammation. But such misadventures, however trying, are not to be compared with trigeminal neuralgia. Nevertheless, in all cases it is the sensory nerve which conducts to the brain the impulse that is eventually translated into the sensation we call pain.

All three sensory branches of the fifth nerve meet in a part of the brain called the 'Gasserian ganglion'. The 'ganglia', of which this is one, may be described as nerve-junctions; a number of them exist for the purpose, as it were, of canalizing through a single department various outlying stations. This grouping takes place on the way to the central receiving station, where the messages will be interpreted as sensations. Now from what has been said it will be obvious that we can abolish pain in several ways. We can interrupt, anywhere along its length, the nerve which is carrying the impulse— this is equivalent to cutting an electric cable. We can break it off where it joins the Gasserian ganglion—this is like pruning the unwanted branch of a tree. Or we can obliterate the ganglion itself—this may be compared either to digging up a plant by the roots or blowing up a junction-box. Any of these methods may be employed, and each has its advantages and drawbacks.

Usually we effect the interruption of the trigeminal nerve by injecting it with alcohol, a process which kills the cells at the desired point. This gives complete relief from pain for a long time; but as the nerve can regenerate itself, further injections may be needed. Absolutely permanent relief is obtained by cutting through the roots of the nerves where they join the ganglion. An advantage of this method is that we can select for treatment whichever of the three branches of the fifth nerve is the one concerned, for as each branch serves a different part of the face, only one may be affected. Lastly, if we wish to abolish the sensory function of all three branches, we can either cut out the ganglion entirely or destroy it, as we do individual nerves, by means of alcohol injection. Nowadays, the operation most favoured is division of the roots of the nerve-branches.

Although these operations at once remove the intolerable pain, they do not touch the part of the body apparently affected. This demonstrates the statement with which the article began—pain is felt, not where we believe we feel it, but in the brain.

HAEMOPHILIA

THE plot of an excellent modern detective story hinges on the exact time when a murder was committed. When the corpse is found lying in a pool of liquid blood, it is concluded that the crime took place only a very short time before the discovery. But this conclusion is wrong—the murder was committed hours earlier; the blood had remained liquid because the victim had suffered from haemophilia, a disease in which blood-coagulation is absent or very long delayed.

What is this disease? Is it common? How do you get it? Can anything be done about it? First we must consider why blood clots at all; why it does not remain permanently liquid; why a cut ever stops bleeding. Blood, as you will have gathered from earlier articles in this book, is not a simple fluid. It is a highly complex aggregation of organic particles floating in a medium which is itself of great complexity. In short, blood is not an ordinary body-fluid, it is really a liquid tissue. If we are wounded severely and blood pours out through a large aperture, we rapidly bleed to death. But we are often wounded slightly, we cut ourselves with tools and implements; thorns scratch us; insects bite us and draw blood. Clearly it would not do if our very lives were threatened by such trivial mishaps. Were there not some automatic safeguard, primitive man could not have survived the hazards of everyday life, and the whole race of mankind would have faded out in the dawn of prehistory.

There is such a safeguard in two substances found in the ordinary blood circulating in the body. These are 'pro-thrombin' and 'fibrinogen'. When blood is shed, the pro-thrombin in the blood near the wound changes to another substance, 'thrombin' (from a Greek word meaning 'clot'). The thrombin then acts upon the fibrinogen in the blood near the wound, converting it into 'fibrin', an insoluble sub-stance. The fibrin forms threads which combine physically with any debris present in the wound, such as broken-down tissues and certain blood-cells, to form a kind of matted plug which we call the clot. When we apply a dressing to a small wound, we help this process; but the essential factor in stopping the loss of blood is its own power of coagulation.

There are some unfortunate people in whose blood this power to coagulate is lacking. We do not know precisely what has gone wrong with the normal mechanism of blood-clotting in them, but strangely enough we do know why. The science of genetics teaches us that inheritable biological characters are transmitted from one generation to another through 'genes', elements in the cells from which all organ-ized bodies grow. Genes from both parents (and, indeed, from all their ancestors) establish the children's attributes, which, as we all know, sometimes resemble closely and some-times differ very widely from the parents'. This, of course, is an over-simplified presentation of an extremely complicated subject. Let us for the moment say, briefly, that a genetic and therefore an inherited defect is responsible for deficient blood-clotting.

Now although this condition is undoubtedly inherited, it is handed down in a very curious way—by the method known as 'sex-linked inheritance'. The simplest means of explaining this term is to describe the actual working of the process. A man has haemophilia. He marries and has both sons and daughters, none of them apparently suffering from their father's complaint. If his sons marry, all their children will be normal, and so will be their succeeding generations for all time. But if one of his daughters marries and has children, her girls will not show haemophilia, but at least some of her boys will—just like their maternal grandfather. And her daughters, though they do not manifest the disease themselves, will transmit it to their sons, just as their mother did. It should be noted that, although we began this pedigree with a haemophiliac man, it is not at all necessary for the transmission of the disease that girls should marry men so affected. If the girl is a 'carrier' of this particular gene (which she will herself have received through her own mother), she will have haemophiliac sons even though her husband is normal. The rule is: manifestation in male offspring, transmission through female.

Haemophilia is quite a serious disease. The tendency to bleed uncontrollably on slight provocation makes even the smallest injury dangerous. The extraction of a tooth, for example, becomes a major operation; a trifling cut or scratch causes greater loss of blood than does a bayonet wound in normal people. A very distressing complication arises when there is bleeding into the cavity of a joint such as the elbow, the ankle, or the knee. The joint swells up and becomes very painful, and afterwards stiffens and hampers movement so that permanent crippling often results.

Because it is a 'family' disease, we may expect haemophilia to be perpetuated more especially in those families where marriages often take place between persons closely related by blood. This was the case in certain European royal families who ruled before the First World War, and the course of history has probably been altered thereby on a number of occasions. There is nothing we can do about haemophilia except to discourage the marriage of girls known to belong to haemophiliac families. This seems a little hard on the girls, but it will be remembered that, even if a haemophiliac man marries a normal woman, all his immediate progeny will be apparently normal (his sons being actually so), and only his daughters can transmit the disease to future heirs. If haemophiliacs had sons only, the disease would die out in a single generation.

FOOD POISONING

THIS common expression is a little indefinite, including several possibilities. Obviously, food may be poisoned by the deliberate addition of some noxious substance, as the Borgias' reputation confirms. Again it may be contaminated 'chemically' either by its containing vessel, or cooking utensil, or literally by accident—something unpleasant falling into it. But 'food poisoning' usually denotes the consequences of consuming food or drink containing something of natural origin injurious to health, and it is to this meaning I shall adhere.

Even so, we must still sub-classify a little. Everyone knows that certain natural products—which in one way or another come to be consumed—are potentially poisonous. For example, nightshade berries contain the poison 'atropine'; some fungi (often mistaken for mushrooms) contain very deadly toxins; rye-flour can be contaminated with 'ergot' (a disease of the grain), with poisonous effects often wrongly suggesting an epidemic, as recently happened on the Continent. Some fish—particularly shellfish—are poisonous, either invariably or at certain seasons, or because they have become infected with disease-germs. But after we have excluded all these kinds of 'food poisoning', we are left with the kind to which the expression should technically be assigned—that caused by the presence of bacteria which have grown in the food at some stage of its preparation, or by the 'toxins' produced by these organisms. Incidentally, some specific diseases can be conveyed in certain foods—for example, tuberculosis in milk and cholera in water. Moreover, conditions such as dysentery and typhoid are associated with the taking of food and drink. But none of these can properly be regarded as examples of food 'poisoning' unless we interpret the word very widely.

Two entirely distinct bacterial agents chiefly cause food poisoning in the restricted sense we have agreed on. One of them which causes the condition called 'botulism', is named *Clostridium botulinum* (after *botulus* = sausage—once supposed to be a special source of disease). Botulism is not only the severest kind of food poisoning, but is one of the most fatal conditions known. Happily it is also one of the rarest; but there have been a number of cases in Britain in recent years: on one occasion eight people who had partaken of the infected food were all dead within a week. Botulism has few premonitory symptoms, sometimes not even any abdominal discomfort, vomiting, or the like. The poison goes straight for the brain where it attacks the cranial nerves, so that the victim's first complaint may be of 'seeing double' within twenty-four hours of being attacked. Then all the nerves are paralysed in turn: swallowing becomes difficult, speech fails, respiration becomes laboured, and death follows—perhaps in as little as thirty-six hours after the entry of the germ, perhaps in a matter of days. All the time the patient is fully conscious and has no pain. At least 50 per cent. of the victims die thus. There is no effective treatment except the injection of an antitoxin, but, as this must be done at a very early stage, all depends on the condition being diagnosed quickly.

After this surfeit of horror it is almost an anti-climax to turn to the other cause of bacterial food poisoning, the *Salmonella* group of organisms. The name has nothing to do with fish but derives from Salmon, the pathologist who first described the group. This large group, consisting of about 150 different types of organism, is responsible for most of the conditions which are diagnosed as food poisoning. True, there are some other organisms outside the group which account for a minority of attacks, but we may take it that three-quarters of all cases of food poisoning are due to Salmonella infection. Members of the Salmonella group may contaminate almost any kind of food, but they have a particular predilection for meat and meat products. 'Processed' meat, such as that used in sausages, meat pies, potted products, and the like, is especially favourable to the growth of these bacteria. Tinned meat, on the contrary, is free from them, though it can, of course, be contaminated after the tin has been opened. Milk also is a common vehicle of Salmonella. Since these bacteria, like the majority of micro-organisms, are very common and widely distributed, it is easy for them to be conveyed to food. Probably most cases of Salmonella infection are attributable to some defect of hygiene in the handling of the food, a defect which may occur at any stage between the farm and the table. Warm weather, delay in serving-up 'left-overs', the presence of house-flies, all these and many other factors encourage the dissemination and growth of the organism. A factor which ought to be non-existent, but is indeed not uncommon, is the contamination of food by the excrement of rats and mice. These animals frequently harbour Salmonella in their bodies, and they are very likely to get at improperly stored food, whether in shops or houses.

There is a general resemblance between the symptoms of all kinds of food poisoning caused by Salmonella. The condition produced, which may be, and usually is, described as 'gastro-enteritis', is an inflammation of the lining of the stomach and the intestines. It comes on within a few hours—twenty-four at the outside—of infection. The first symptom is usually a feeling of nausea, or as some people call it 'sick headache'. A bout of diarrhoea, perhaps accompanied by pain in the abdomen, follows and continues for two or three days, when the attack passes off. Normally it is only a minor illness, but occasionally a more serious form develops in which the victim suffers from a kind of fever—in some respects not unlike typhoid—for a week or more. There are even more serious forms, happily rare, which end fatally. Treatment, which is mainly directed towards the relief of the pain, diarrhoea, &c., includes rest in bed and a liquid diet. Recently the antibiotic 'chloramphenicol' has been used to attack the Salmonella directly, and the sulpha drugs 'sulphasuxidine' and 'sulphaguanidine' have been found valuable. Prevention is of course achieved by the strictest observance of hygiene in the handling of all food and drink. Unfortunately, this cannot be guaranteed everywhere along the line which connects producer with consumer, but at least we can each do our part. Though there may be no noticeable sign that food or milk is 'bad', no unpleasant odour or the like, it may nevertheless contain Salmonella organisms, for these are not related to decomposition at all. Food sufficiently advanced in decomposition to be poisonous would be obviously uneatable.

Perhaps at this point I should say a word about 'ptomaine

poisoning'. There really is no such thing, for practical purposes. The complex organic compounds known as ptomaines
are indeed poisonous in their way (though not as a rule
when swallowed—they need to be injected), but they are
found only in substances which have reached an advanced
state of decomposition. And however great one's liking for
'high' food, it must be so exceptional a palate that enjoys
something actually putrefying, that the risk of 'ptomaine
poisoning' is practically negligible. The expression was
coined before the bacterial nature of food poisoning was
understood.

ALLERGY

Our language affords many instances of the perversion of
words from their original meanings. A recent example is the
everyday use of the word 'allergic', which formerly had a
strictly technical significance. We now say that we are allergic to a certain thing or person when we mean that we are
averse to it or him. But the two words are not at all synonymous. In medical science, an allergic individual is one
whose body reacts in an abnormal way to the introduction
of certain substances, often very common substances which
do no harm to most people. Usually very minute quantities
of the 'allergen' evoke the abnormal reaction, with striking
disproportion between cause and effect.

This state of allergy shows itself in several ways, producing results so various that it is difficult to believe they are
manifestations of the same thing. One of the most distressing
of human complaints to experience or to witness is asthma.
In a typical attack, the sufferer has great difficulty in
breathing—he feels suffocated, he gasps painfully, his every
breath is accompanied by a loud 'wheeze', his face turns

purple, the veins in his neck stand out, and his body breaks into a sweat. Frequently, it is allergy which causes asthma.

Then there is hay fever, a disorder which is regarded rather facetiously by everyone except its victims. It produces the symptoms of streaming eyes and nose, violent sneezing, and general symptoms of severe catarrh, which come upon them inevitably at certain seasons of the year. Here again the principal agent is allergy.

A very different disorder, which no one would think related to these two, is 'urticaria' or nettlerash. This is a skin eruption—'wheals' suddenly appear over various areas of the body, intolerably irritating while they last. Fortunately they do not usually last very long; but there is a kind of nettlerash in which as one crop of itchy patches dies away a fresh outbreak takes its place. This condition can become chronic. Allergy again is the culprit.

There is some doubt whether 'angio-neurotic oedema' is truly a kind of nettlerash, though it is often termed the 'giant' variety. As the latter name implies, big swellings occur, usually much bigger than those described above. Frequently these swellings affect the face—commonly the lips and the eyelids—but they can occur anywhere. If they come up inside the mouth or throat, as they do sometimes, the victim may die of suffocation in a matter of minutes. Perhaps not every case of angio-neurotic oedema is due to allergy, but many undoubtedly are.

There are a number of other conditions for which allergy is possibly to blame: the very severe kind of headache called migraine, some forms of skin diseases (other than those noted above), a particular kind of chronic cold in the head, and a number of occupational maladies, one associated with bee-keeping. Even some kinds of rheumatism, and of stomach and bowel disturbances, may be of allergic origin.

We said at the beginning that allergic reactions are

provoked when certain substances are taken into the body. First it should be understood that it is immaterial how these 'allergens' get in—they may be swallowed, or inhaled, or applied to the skin—the result to a 'sensitive' person is the same. There is the widest imaginable range of them. High on the list come certain kinds of dust (notably grass-pollens), animal hairs, eggs, strawberries, oysters, feathers, and face-powders. But as a rule a person is sensitive to only one particular allergen; it is as if his constitutional reaction were kept in a locked compartment which only one key can open.

All allergens have one thing in common—they all have the composition of 'proteins', those very complex substances which are found normally in animal and plant tissues. We need some proteins in our diet, but some are, to the individual sufferer from allergy, 'foreign' proteins, substances not normal to his body. The mechanism by which the allergic reaction is brought about is exceedingly complicated and cannot be described at length. We must be content here to accept the fact that some people, after taking into the body certain foreign proteins, release in their tissues a substance called 'histamine'. This is a naturally occurring compound, but for our present purpose it must be regarded as a poison, and we can show by experiment that it is responsible for all the effects of allergy.

When a person suffering from some allergic complaint seeks medical advice, the doctors will try to find his specific allergen—just what it is which provokes his symptoms. This can be a very long job, and sometimes they never do discover the offensive material. But there is usually something to go on, so that by a process of elimination it can often be tracked down. The equipment of a doctor who specializes in this kind of detective work includes a vast array of little phials each containing different allergen extracts ranging from essence of eiderdown to shellfish-juice! A series of these is applied to a small area of the patient's skin. If the investigator is lucky, before he has gone very far he finds something to which the patient's skin gives the typical allergic reaction. If he is unlucky, he may have to work through the entire series.

If this evidence points to a definite allergen—if, so to speak, the criminal's fingerprints are identified—cure may be attempted by 'desensitization'. This method consists of giving the patient a number of injections of small doses of his special allergen, in the hope that he will thereby acquire immunity—the principle is similar to that which operates in other forms of immunization against disease. Of course, if the allergen is discovered to be an article of food, the treatment, or rather prevention, is simply to abstain from that food.

Of late a method has come into use which depends on a different principle. We have seen that the essential feature of all allergic disorders is the release of histamine in the tissues. Now it is quite logical to use an antidote to neutralize a poison, and a number of antidotes to histamine have been found. Some can be swallowed, some are injected, some inhaled. They act by antagonizing the action of the liberated histamine—some perhaps by preventing its release. The administration of anti-histamines does not abolish the patient's constitutional tendency to allergic reactions—the anti-histamines deal effectually with the attack, but they are not preventives. This method does not attempt to cure the underlying condition as desensitization does.

Although it is not, strictly speaking, relevant to our subject, it may here be mentioned that various anti-histamine drugs have been advocated as cures for the common cold. It will be apparent that they cannot be a general remedy, their efficacy is confined to cases involving some degree of allergy. And however closely the symptoms of hay fever may appear to resemble those of a severe cold, they spring from an entirely different cause, and it is unsafe to conclude that the treatment for the one is proper for the other.

CONCLUSION

I HAVE tried to recount in simple language something of the story of human illness, how it is caused and what can be done to relieve it. We do not yet know the whole story, though each instalment brings its end nearer. And what a wonderful story it is. There is no comparison between the state of world health today and that of a century ago. The astonishing progress of medical science has benefited not a single privileged class or race, but all mankind. The fever-racked peasant of a backward country is restored to health no less than the diabetic citizen of a highly civilized community. Our knowledge, however, is still imperfect in many important respects, and too often the conquest of older diseases is accompanied by the uprising of new ills. Tuberculosis wanes but cancer increases; fewer are crippled in body but many more are disturbed in mind. Still, the great task goes forward. Every passing year enables us to say of some sufferer, 'Not long ago he would have died.'

In such a book as this only a bare outline of its vast subject can be attempted, only fundamental aspects described. Nor can more than a very few of the five thousand or so officially recognized diseases be even mentioned. Those that I have selected for mention are of special interest, because of their general importance, because they typify some basic principle of causation or treatment, or because they present problems cognate to others already solved. Thus it happens that a comparatively rare condition like trigeminal neuralgia receives notice along with an exceedingly common one like arthritis, and the fatal leukaemias are given almost as much attention as an eminently curable disease like malaria. Minor accidents like sprained joints are—in order to illustrate a principle—considered, along with apoplexy, which illustrates another.

Although the structure of this book is avowedly pathological, its bases are anatomy and physiology. Naturally, some conditions more than others demand accounts of the normal features of structure and function, for example, thrombosis, thyroid diseases, hypertension, anaemia. But I have wished to stress, in all cases, that some acquaintance with the normal is essential to an understanding of the abnormal. More, I have purposed to show that the very complicated process of human disease can be analysed, as it were, into a comparatively few component stages; that effects presenting little outward similarity stem from similar causes, and equally that greatly differing causes can produce like effects. I asked my readers in the introductory article to regard the book as a whole, to discover for themselves its pattern. I should like, in these concluding words, briefly to recapitulate the themes. We have spoken of diseases transmitted by four different kinds of micro-organisms, 'bacteria', 'protozoa', 'viruses', and 'rickettsias'; we have considered examples of 'vector-borne' diseases as well as those conveyed by direct contagion; and have recognized those which select individuals and those which tend to run in epidemics. We have described other conditions not due to infection by living agents, for example the endocrine diseases and the anaemias. We have studied inherited states like haemophilia; constitutional affections like allergy; diseases of doubtful causation like hypertension. We have recounted what is known of malignant disease. We have described the disorders of the special senses which cause deafness and blindness, and said something of mental disorder. We have not utterly neglected 'surgical' cases, some of them being mentioned in the articles on dislocations, fractures, and hernia. For the interest of those who may have encountered them overseas, we have included an all-too-brief survey of a very few of the more important 'tropical' diseases.

This book not only recounts the victories of the past and reports the struggles of today, but expresses the lively hope that evils as yet impregnable will in time be added to the list of citadels overthrown by medicine. In the pursuit of that end science and art join hands; the study and practice of medicine is one of the noblest of human endeavours, its history glorified by acts of heroism and self-abnegation. Perhaps some readers of this humble tribute may be encouraged to join those who carry the standard forward in that unceasing war of humanity. There is work crying out to be done, and it must be so for generations, perhaps centuries. Shall we not have for our generation, our century, the epitaph of an ancient cause:

> *'The stubborn spearmen still made good*
> *Their dark impenetrable wood:*
> *Each stepping where his comrade stood,*
> *The instant that he fell.'*

INDEX

PRINTED IN
GREAT BRITAIN
AT THE
UNIVERSITY PRESS
OXFORD
BY
CHARLES BATEY
PRINTER
TO THE
UNIVERSITY